AURAL REHABILITATION FOR PEOPLE WITH DISABILITIES

AURAL REHABILITATION FOR PEOPLE WITH DISABILITIES

John M.A. Oyiborhoro
Boro Audiology Clinic
Brooklyn, New York
and
National Institute for People with Disabilities
New York, New York

ELSEVIER
ACADEMIC
PRESS

AMSTERDAM • BOSTON • HEIDELBERG • LONDON
NEW YORK • OXFORD • PARIS • SAN DIEGO
SAN FRANCISCO • SINGAPORE • SYDNEY • TOKYO

Elsevier Academic Press
30 Corporate Drive, Suite 400, Burlington, MA 01803, USA
525 B Street, Suite 1900, San Diego, California 92101-4495, USA
84 Theobald's Road, London WC1X 8RR, UK

This book is printed on acid-free paper. ∞

Library of Congress Cataloging-in-Publication Data
Application submitted

British Library Cataloguing in Publication Data
A catalogue record for this book is available from the British Library

ISBN: 0-12-531785-9

For all information on all Elsevier Academic Press publications
visit our website at www.books.elsevier.com

Printed in the United States of America
05   06   07   08   09   9   8   7   6   5   4   3   2   1

To Parents and Direct Caregivers of People with Severe Disabilities
and
To Onakpoma (Ono) for Her Love, Support, and Motherly Care

CONTENTS

CHAPTER 1
Overview of Disabilities
John M.A. Oyiborhoro, Ed.D., F.A.A.A., CCC-A

PART I
Audiologic Rehabilitation for People with Disabilities: Assessment and Management

CHAPTER 2
Cerebral Palsy/Developmental Disabilities
John M.A. Oyiborhoro, Ed.D., F.A.A.A., CCC-A

CHAPTER 3
HIV/AIDS

John M.A. Oyiborhoro, Ed.D., F.A.A.A., CCC-A

CHAPTER 4
People with Visual Impairment

Cindy Gustin, PH, MSc

CHAPTER 5

Older Adults with Dementia or Alzheimer's Disease

Emi Isaki, Ph.D., CCC/SLP

CHAPTER 9

Augmentative and Alternative Communication

Mary Jean J. Dyczko, M.A., CCC/SLP, TSHH, ATP and
Nancy Lenhart Jones, M.S., CCC/SLP, TSHH, ATP

CHAPTER 10

RESPECTFUL Counseling: A Blueprint for Practice

Brenda Y. Cartwright, Ed.D., CRC, LPC

CONTRIBUTORS

Numbers in parentheses indicate the pages on which the authors' contributions begin.

Brenda Y. Cartwright, Ed.D., CRC, LPC (287), Department of Counselor Education, University of Hawaii at Manoa, Honolulu, HA

Mary Jean J. Dyczko, M.A., CCC/SLP, TSHH, ATP (210), NYS Licensed Speech-Language Pathologist, RESNA Certified Assistive Technology Practitioner, Practicing Augmentative and Alternative Communication Specialist, New York, NY

Cindy Gustin, PH, MSc (79), St. Paul's Hospital, Vancouver, British Columbia

Emi Isaki, Ph.D., CCC/SLP (118), Division of Speech Pathology and Audiology, John A. Burns School of Medicine, University of Hawaii at Manoa, Honolulu, HA

Nancy Lenhart Jones, M.S., CCC/SLP, TSHH, ATP (210), NYS Licensed Speech-Language Pathologist, RESNA Certified Assistive Technology Practitioner, Practicing Augmentative and Alternative Communication Specialist, New York, NY

Gita J. Malur, M.D. (134), Pediatric Healthcare Unlimited, Alton, IL

John M.A. Oyiborhoro, Ed.D., F.A.A.A., CCC-A (1, 26, 59, 154), Boro Audiology Clinic, Brooklyn, NY; National Institute for People with Disabilities, New York, NY

Teralandur K. Parthasarathy, Ph.D. (134), Department of Special Education and Communication Disorders, Southern Illinois University Edwardsville, Edwardsville, IL

Kenneth C. Pugh, Ph.D. (174), Division of Speech Pathology and Audiology, John A. Burns School of Medicine, University of Hawaii at Manoa, Honolulu, HA

FOREWORD

During the 1940s audiology was established by its founders as a profession that provided aural rehabilitation for GIs newly deafened in World War II. From this important beginning, audiology experienced a broad expansion of its scope of practice from identification of hearing loss in the newborn to diagnostic assessment of site of lesion in the auditory system. At this time many audiologists provide aural rehabilitation to children and adults in pediatric settings, schools, community clinics, dispensing audiology practices, and other venues. Nevertheless, in many ways aural rehabilitation has not received the focus of professional attention that is deserved by the persons we serve.

This timely book takes us back to our roots and reminds us about the importance and place of aural rehabilitation for persons with a wide range of disabilities. Dr. Oyiborhoro has assembled a panel of knowledgeable authors to explore the problems of assessment and management of individuals with unique and sometimes devastating diseases. The topics include several areas of discussion including amplification and assistive technology, augmentative and alternative communication, and the important area of counseling.

Readers of this book will find the information to be helpful as they provide services to people with disabilities. The information is applicable to a wide range of readers from students to experienced practicing audiologists. Speech-language pathologists and others who work with hearing-impaired persons who have other disabilities will also find this book to be an important resource.

I congratulate Dr. Oyiborhoro for his efforts in bringing this important project to fruition. I am sure that the readers will join me in their appreciation of the information provided here.

Robert W. Keith, Ph.D.
Professor and Director
Division of Audiology and Vestibular Testing
University of Cincinnati Medical Center
Cincinnati, Ohio USA

July 21, 2004

ACKNOWLEDGMENTS

The impetus for writing this book was provided while working with the wonderful consumers (people with special needs) at the United Cerebral Palsy of New York City, Inc.; the National Institute for People with Disabilities, also known as YAI; Heartshare Wellness; the Hebrew Academy for Special Children (HASC); and Bais Ezra in New York. I am grateful to the consumers, their parents, their significant others, and their direct caregivers for teaching me so much about patience, love, endurance, wisdom, and appreciation for human life. I thank my colleagues at the United Cerebral Palsy of New York City, Inc., especially David Gross, Anthony Aversano, and Mrs. Miriam Pratt for their support and friendship.

My special thanks to my teachers at Teachers College, Columbia University in New York City and at Case Western Reserve University in Cleveland, Ohio, especially Drs. Barbara Weinstein, Craig Newman, Hugh Catts, and Celia Hooper. I am grateful to Mrs. Valenta Ward-Gravely for imparting her incisive clinical skills and to Professor James Nation and Drs. Danielle Ripich and Alex F. Johnson for their understanding and support. Also, I thank Donald and Debbie Robin for the shared and rewarding experiences at Case Western Reserve University. The assistance of my former students at Pace University in New York City in the initial literature search and references is appreciated. My thanks to Dr. Dorothy Ogundu for her constant reminders and encouragement to complete the book, and to Drs. George Mencher and Ross J. Roeser for their interest and support. I wish to thank Rebecca Ann Conrow, Ari Abreau, Genni Arreaga, Adriana Rua, and Lola Pearson for their help. My special thanks to my family for their support and encouragement. I also extend my thanks to the former and present staff of Academic Press, especially Mark Zadrozny for the initial contacts and Mara Conner for her patience, understanding, and encouragement in completing the book.

John M.A. Oyiborhoro

CHAPTER 1

Overview of Disabilities

John M.A. Oyiborhoro, Ed.D., F.A.A.A., CCC-A
Boro Audiology Clinic
Brooklyn, NY
and
National Institute for People with Disabilities
New York, NY

Concept of Disability
Consequences of Hearing Impairment
Mental Retardation
Down's Syndrome
Cerebral Palsy
HIV/AIDS
Visual Impairment
Sociocultural Issues
Management of People with Disabilities
People with Other Disabilities
References
Selected Readings

The Americans with Disabilities Act was enacted into law in 1990. The law required that equal opportunities be created by employers for individuals with any form of disability. Any form of discrimination, especially in employment, was prohibited by the new law. Since then significant changes have been made in places of employment, entertainment, and education to actualize this new law of inclusion. To enhance communication, public facilities, where necessary, are required to provide auxiliary devices for individuals with hearing, vision, or speech impairments. Auxiliary devices include assistive listening devices, television captioning and decoders, telecommunication devices for the deaf (TDD), video text displays, reader taped texts, and brailled materials as well as large-print materials.

The Developmental Disabilities Assistance and Bill of Rights Act of 1990 defined developmental disability as a severe, chronic disability of an individual 5 years of age or older that is

1. attributable to a mental or physical impairment or a combination of both;
2. manifested before the individual attains age 22;
3. likely to continue indefinitely; and
4. likely to result in substantial functional limitations in **three** or more of the following areas of major life activity such as (i) self-care, (ii) receptive and expressive language, (iii) learning, (iv) mobility, (v) self-direction, (vi) capacity for independent living, (vii) economic self-sufficiency, and (viii) demonstration of "the individual's need for a combination and sequence of special interdisciplinary or genetic services, support, or other assistance that are of lifelong or extended duration and are individually planned and coordinated. . . ." (p. 1192)

Developmental disabilities do not usually occur in isolation. In many cases, disabilities may be present in the same individual but in varying degrees. For instance, a person with cerebral palsy (CP) may have normal or near-normal intelligence or may present a severe degree of mental retardation, may be verbal or nonverbal, and/or may also have a hearing loss. Similarly, an individual with Down's syndrome may be nonverbal with hearing loss, mental retardation, and some autistic features. Other individuals may have a hearing loss and also present visual impairment and some behavioral problems. The presence of other disabilities in the same individual, no matter how minor or mild, tends to magnify the impact of the primary disability. For instance, take the case of an individual who has a mild degree of mental retardation. The presence of an unidentified and untreated hearing loss in this individual is likely to make the mental retardation appear worse than it actually is. Depending on the degree and extent of occurrence, developmental disabilities pose significant handicaps for affected individuals, and these often can have an impact on their quality of life. The goal of aural rehabilitation of these individuals is to provide audiologic evaluation and ways by which the consequences of the handicaps caused by these disabilities can be ameliorated through the use of hearing amplification, augmentative communication, and appropriate referrals.

CONCEPT OF DISABILITY

The terms disability, handicap, and impairment are often used or misused interchangeably in rehabilitation literature. *Disability* refers to a physical, physiologic, mental, or sensory abnormality, whereas *handicap* refers to the consequences caused by the disability. A handicap is the extent and degree to which a disability impedes, limits, or restricts an individual's participation in certain activities or tasks for which a normal body function is needed. Disability therefore results in activity limitation or participation restriction as a result of the presence of a physical or physiologic dysfunction that an individual may present. The World Health Organization (1980) defines an *impairment* as any loss or abnormality of psychologic, physiologic, or anatomical structure or function. The degree to which an impairment poses a handicap is a function of the extent and degree of the impairment itself. Impairment relates to disability in that both occur as a result of loss of function of an anatomical or physiologic nature that limits activity or restricts the individual's participation. Hearing loss, for instance, causes activity limitation (disability) and social/occupational participation restriction (handicap).

Hearing loss is an invisible disability that affects people of any age group from neonates to older adults. Hearing impairment of any degree or configuration is capable of compromising communication, education, social functioning, and safety of the individual. The evaluation and management of hearing loss, particularly in infants and young and older adults, can be challenging. However, there is yet another group of people who, apart from having hearing deficits, present additional disabilities, disease processes, or dysfunctions that sometimes further compromise the hearing loss itself. However, such additional disease processes or conditions may be primary, secondary, or totally unrelated to a hearing loss. These problematic conditions may be developmental such as mental retardation, Down's syndrome, cerebral palsy, and autism; may be related to a disease process such as human immunodeficiency virus infection (HIV)/acquired immunodeficiency syndrome (AIDS) and other conditions that can cause the disruption of auditory or visual function, physical motor function, or sensory motor function; or may be disorders in speech, language, and cognition.

Despite rapid advancement in medicine, science, and technology, the number of people with disabilities has not yet decreased significantly. Natural occurrences due to chromosome defects as well as to pre, peri, and postnatal events and traumatic accidents during delivery have contributed to the numbers of people with disabilities in our society. It is also possible that we now have better methods of detecting and describing new human developmental problems and disease processes. Some good examples of discoveries of new conditions are AIDS and severe acute respiratory syndrome (SARS). It is simply not possible to be familiar with every known disability. In addition, many times clinicians do not feel they possess adequate training or skills to evaluate hearing-impaired people with other more commonly encountered disabilities, such as CP, visual impairment, mental retardation, dementia, and Down's syndrome. These disabilities may be primary to, secondary to, or even unrelated to hearing impairment. Very young and elderly individuals pose greater challenges for audiologic evaluations and rehabilitation, especially if other disabilities are present. Usually, a diagnosis of the dominant disability is important. Based on this diagnosis, specific audiologic test batteries can be selected.

For instance, the HIV/AIDS epidemic has occurred during the past two decades. The literature is replete with reports of structural damage and loss of function resulting from the impact of HIV/AIDS on the auditory system (Grimaldi, et al., 1993; Moazzez & Alvin, 1998; Pappas, Roland, Lim, Lai, & Hillman, 1995; Soucek & Michael, 1996). New disease processes and conditions as exemplified by the recent SARS epidemic will continue to emerge even with advancements in sophisticated diagnostic and therapeutic methods in science and medicine to address known and unknown pathologic conditions. Some of these pathologic conditions may occur as handicaps that are primary to or associated with hearing impairment. Associated or dominant handicaps in hearing-impaired individuals may sometimes delay the diagnosis of hearing impairment (Voutilainen, Jauhiainen, & Linkola, 1998). Until recently hearing impairment was often not thought to be crucial in the initial evaluation of children with disabilities, because it was not considered a priority in the overall rehabilitation process (Friedrich, 1985). However, in the United States, this attitude is changing now that universal neonatal hearing screening programs are in place in many states. In these states, a hearing screening test is performed on every neonate before discharge from the hospital. In addition, noninvasive and more objective tools such as otoacoustic emissions and auditory brainstem response are now in common use.

However, although these objective electrophysiologic tests generally yield a more accurate status of auditory function than previously used methods, they also have pitfalls (Worthington & Peters, 1980). With behavioral assessment measures still being widely used, many individuals with associated handicaps may still be considered to be untestable, especially when clinicians are either uncomfortable or unfamiliar with a dominant disability and its effects on hearing function and the evaluation process. Some of these disabilities will be discussed briefly later.

CONSEQUENCES OF HEARING IMPAIRMENT

Because hearing impairment is an invisible disability, it is easily ignored, especially if other, more dominant, health issues are also present. If hearing impairment, whether mild or unilateral, is not identified early enough—either at birth or within the first 2 years of life—it may have serious consequences for the child's speech, language, and cognitive skills development. The child's educational process and achievement may also be compromised if a hearing loss is unidentified and rehabilitation is not instituted. In the United States, as noted earlier, neonatal hearing screening is now common in many states. Neonates usually receive routine screening to rule out the presence of a hearing loss before their discharge from the hospital after delivery. An infant with suspected hearing loss is followed, and appropriate diagnostic and rehabilitative measures are put in place. However, for children with multiple disabilities, the presence of a hearing loss, its evaluation, and rehabilitation constitute additional challenges.

MENTAL RETARDATION

Audiologic evaluation, particularly the behavioral aspect, is an interactive process. The clinician and the individual being tested must interact communicatively with each other to obtain accurate hearing thresholds. This interaction requires a minimal level of intellectual functioning and adaptive abilities for an individual to respond appropriately to speech and acoustic stimuli. Chromosomal abnormalities, heredity, pre- and perinatal infections, intrauterine growth retardation, and inappropriate or indiscriminate exposure of the fetus to drugs during pregnancy are common causes of mental retardation. Socioeconomic factors such as poor nutrition, maternal neglect, and poverty can compound preexisting low intellectual function. Although there is some disagreement concerning the use of the term *mental retardation*, there is unanimity that an individual with this condition must exhibit low intellectual functioning, an impairment due to physical insult, disease, or an abnormality before age 18, and an impairment in adaptive abilities (Batshaw and Shapiro, 1997). IQ scores, age of onset, and adaptive impairments (although still controversial) have often been used to define mental retardation. According to the American Psychiatric Association (1994), a person with mental retardation should exhibit the following characteristics: an IQ score of 70 or less on an individually administered IQ test, concurrent deficits in adaptive functioning, and onset before the age of 18 years. Impairment in adaptive ability is demonstrated by the person's inability to perform at least two culturally expected and age-appropriate skills required for everyday living such as communication, self-care, social/interpersonal skills, functional academic skills, home living, safe use of community resources, and self-direction in work, leisure activities, and health. Some of the everyday living skills that are vital during audiologic evaluation and rehabilitation are easily compromised by more severe mental retardation. For instance, a person with mild mental retardation (IQ score of approximately 70) would perform much better on speech measures that require repeating words or sentences than an individual with severe retardation (IQ score of approximately 35).

DOWN'S SYNDROME

Down's syndrome is caused by three types of chromosomal abnormalities: trisomy 21, translocation, and mosaicism. People with Down's syndrome often have craniofacial anomalies and are prone to having pathologic conditions of the middle ear, especially Eustachian tube dysfunction. Hearing impairment occurs in about 60–80% of individuals with Down's syndrome (MCW Health Link; 2002; Roizen, Wolters, Nicol, & Blondis, 1993), who exhibit various degrees and types of hearing impairment. Although the hearing loss can be sensorineural, conductive, or mixed conductive, conductive hearing loss is the most commonly occurring type of hearing loss seen in this group. Smaller and narrow ear canals, which are often impacted with cerumen are common, especially in children. Audiologic management of this group involves a series of audiologic evaluations, medical or surgical intervention, use of amplification, and caregiver education.

CEREBRAL PALSY

CP is a condition, not a disease. *Cerebral palsy* is an umbrella term used to describe disorders of motor function resulting from brain injury or malfunction. Brain injuries that cause CP often may also result in other associated problems such as hearing and vision disorders, mental retardation, and speech and language impairment. CP is associated with two main types of brain injury: spastic (pyramidal) and athetoid (extrapyramidal). The most common form of CP is the spastic type, which is characterized by tense, contracted muscles and limited movements of the head, neck, and limbs. Both forms of CP have implications for audiologic assessment and rehabilitation, especially in terms of selection of test battery, evaluation techniques, testee response modes, hearing instruments, and rehabilitation when indicated.

HIV/AIDS

AIDS is caused by HIV. The disease, first described in 1981, has had devastating effects on health, including the hearing health of those living with AIDS. AIDS gradually and gravely affects the central nervous system (CNS) with substantial manifestations in the head and neck regions of the body in which the auditory system is also extensively represented (Bankaitis & Keith, 1995; Lalwani & Sooy, 1992; Real, Thomas, & Gerwins, 1987; Timon & Walsh, 1989). Thus many HIV-infected individuals often report a triad of vertigo, tinnitus, and hearing loss. However, HIV does not directly produce hearing loss; hearing impairment results from opportunistic infections caused by the manifestation of HIV infection (Rarey, 1990; Wilson, 1986). Otitis media, which is prevalent in this population, is often caused by opportunistic infecting agents secondary to HIV infection (Lalwani & Sooy, 1992). Sensorineural hearing loss also occurs commonly in this population, in part because of heavy reliance on cocktails of experimental and potentially ototoxic antibiotics for the medical management of patients living with HIV.

VISUAL IMPAIRMENT

There are various degrees of visual impairment that are defined by the extent of visual acuity. An individual who has a visual acuity of 20/200 or worse in the better eye with correction or a visual field that is greater than a 20-degree angle is regarded to be *legally blind* (Bishop, 1991). According to the Education for All Handicapped Children Act of 1995 (PL 94-142) and Buncic (1987), partially sighted individuals or individuals with low vision, on the other hand, have a visual acuity that is better than 20/200 but worse than 20/70 with correction. Although some people who are considered legally blind may have sufficient residual vision to be able to identify various objects and colors and read large print, others lack light and dark perception (Menacker & Batshaw, 1997). Visual impairment has considerable implications for the way hearing is evaluated in terms of choice of test materials and method of evaluation and the test environment itself.

Although visual impairment can be a standalone disability, often it occurs in association with other disabilities such as diabetes. Congenital causes of visual impairment commonly are intrauterine infections and malformation of the visual system itself. Infections and other causes of blindness such as brain trauma and anoxia are commonly associated with other disabilities such as hearing impairment, CP, and mental retardation.

Apart from the disorders briefly discussed here, hearing loss is found as a significant component in nearly 400 different syndromes (Schaefer, 1995). Schaefer reported the top 10 syndromes that are most commonly associated with hearing impairment as follows:

1. Hemifacial microsomia
2. Stickler syndrome
3. Congenital cytomegalovirus virus infection
4. Usher's syndrome
5. Branchio-otorenal syndrome
6. Pendred's syndrome
7. CHARGE association
8. Neurofibromatosis type II
9. Mitochondrial disorders
10. Waardenburg syndrome

The incidence, identifying features, types of auditory disorders, and hearing loss that are associated with these syndromes are displayed in Table 1.1.

SOCIOCULTURAL ISSUES

The Americans with Disabilities Act of 1990 mandates accessibility for the hearing impaired as well as for people with other disabilities. Parental beliefs, attitudes, and cultural practices have a great influence on acceptance of their children's disabilities and their motivation to get actively involved in rehabilitation (Danseco, 1997; Mardiros, 1989). For instance, a parent who believes that a child's disability is temporary only and hopes that the child will outgrow the problems (Danseco, 1997) will not be easily persuaded to seek help for his or her child. Some parents believe that the arrival of a handicapped child

Table 1.1
Syndromes Associated with Significant Hearing Loss

Syndrome	Incidence	Common identifying features	Auditory disorders/ hearing loss	Suggestions/comments
1. Hemifacial microsomia (oculoauriculovertebral dysplasia, Goldenhar's syndrome)	Unknown	Facial asymmetry Ocular abnormalities (anophthalmia, micro-ophthalmia, and epibulbar dermoids) Auricular abnormalities (microtia, atresia, anotia) Cervical spine and cranial base malformations	Conductive and/or sensorineural Auricular abnormalities Anomalies of middle and external ears Eustachian tube malformations and dysfunction Cranial nerve and skull cranial base abnormalities	Conduct complete conventional and special tests.
2. Stickler syndrome (Marshall–Stickler syndrome, hereditary arthro–ophthalmopathy)	Unknown	Craniofacial abnormalities Cleft palate Flattening of the face Ocular changes Arthropathy	Conductive hearing loss Progressive sensorineural Eustachian tube dysfunction (caused by cleft palate)	Refer for genetic counseling.
3. Congenital cytomegalovirus infection (CMV)	1 of 3500 live births	Jaundice, hemolytic amnesia, thrombocytopenia, hepatosplenomegaly Microcephaly Cerebral calcifications Central nervous system disruptions	Sensorineural (may be progressive)	Confirm CMV as a cause of hearing loss from serologic and epidemiologic findings

4. Usher's syndrome	3.5 per 100,000 live births	Retinitis pigmentosa Sensorineural loss Absent vestibular function in type I	Moderate to severe sensorineural Severe to profound sensorineural Progressive (in some patients) 10% of individuals with retinitis pigmentosa have hearing loss 10% of children with sensorineural hearing loss have Usher's syndrome	Not all individuals with retinitis pigmentosa and sensor neural hearing loss have Usher's syndrome. Conduct complete audiologic evaluation and electronystagmography (ENG).
5. Branchio–otorenal syndrome (BOR)	1 per 40,000 live births 2% of children with profound hearing loss may have BOR	Branchial clefts Fistulas and cysts Malformation of pinnae Preauricular pits	Significant hearing loss 30% conductive 20% sensorineural 50% Mixed	Refer for special imaging tests to identify renal malformation.
6. Pendred's syndrome	5% of individuals with congenital hearing loss	Thyroid goiter Profound congenital sensorineural hearing loss	Hearing loss often present Severe hearing loss present more than 50% of the time Progressive hearing loss	Test for thyroid integrity and function.
7. CHARGE association	Unknown	Coloboma Heart problems Atresia Retarded growth and development Genital hyperplasia Ear anomaly/deafness (CHARGE)	Mixed hearing loss 80–85% of individuals with CHARGE have hearing loss	Check case history for CHARGE features.

(continues)

Table 1.1

(*Continued*)

Syndrome	Incidence	Common identifying features	Auditory disorders/ hearing loss	Suggestions/comments
8. Neurofibromatosis type II	1 in 40,000 (children) 1 in ≥200,000 (adults)	Vestibular schwannomas Intracranial tumors	Unilateral Progressive	Neurofibromatosis type II may explain noncongenital unilateral hearing impairment. Magnetic resonance imaging (MRI) test suggested.
9. Mitochondrial disorders	Unknown	Hearing loss Seizure disorder Diabetes mellitus Cardiac defects Ataxia Optic atrophy	Sensorineural	Hearing loss is often associated with maternal inheritance
10. Waardenburg syndrome	1 to 4000 live births 2.3% of children with congenital hearing loss	Craniofacial anomalies Multiple pigmentary abnormalities (e.g., white forelock, partial albinism, early graying)	Sensorineural Unilateral or bilateral	None

Adapted from Schaefer, G. B. (1995). Ten syndromes most commonly associated with hearing impairment. *Advances in the genetics of deafness: A Bulletin of the HHIRR, 2*(1) .

into the family is a punishment and an expression of anger from offended gods and a sign of greater misfortunes to come (Oyiborhoro, 1984). In some cultures, the Supreme Being is believed to protect innocent humans from every evil doer, and, furthermore, the gods are also believed to be aware of any fetus that plans evil from the moment of conception. Thus, to prevent such evil plans from materializing, the child is deformed by the gods. In certain societies from which some new American immigrants originate, handicapped children are either destroyed, ignored, exploited, or banished with their families from the community. Some of these belief systems and cultural practices are carried with these immigrants when they arrive in the United States, and they have to cope with reconciling an old, traditional system that they were used to with a new, modernized one. In some traditional societies, religious beliefs encourage the giving and taking of alms in the streets. A handicapped child is considered a blessing, especially in poverty-stricken areas, because this means the arrival of another breadwinner for the family. The more severe a disability is, the better, because the disabled person will be more pitied and cared for by sympathizers and benefactors. Sometimes the conditions of physically disabled children or adults worsen or their conditions are untreated to embellish existing physical defects so they will look more pathetic in the public eye. According to such a belief system, the main goal of the handicapped person is to attract as much alms as possible from benefactors.

America is a multicultural and multiethnic country composed of people with diverse experiences from almost every part of the world. This cultural diversity is increasing. According to the U.S. Bureau of Census (2000) about 80% of new immigrants who arrive in the United States speak a language other than English at home. Audiologic assessment and aural rehabilitation plans should take into consideration cultural backgrounds of handicapped children and their parents to achieve the desired goals. In taking the case history of the individual, for instance, culturally sensitive questions may need to be modified to gather culturally and linguistically relevant data (Ballachanda, 2001). It is important to note that the concept of disability, hearing impairments and the handicap that they pose, acceptance, and even rehabilitation needs vary from culture to culture and also can be viewed very differently.

MANAGEMENT OF PEOPLE WITH DISABILITIES

Aural rehabilitation is a process designed to ameliorate the impact and consequences of hearing impairment. For hearing-impaired people without other disabilities, the goal of aural rehabilitation is primarily the acquisition of spoken speech and language skills. The focus of aural rehabilitation is on how best to maximize the functional use of the patient's residual hearing through use of amplification and appropriate educational plans that facilitate and enhance learning. The success of the *aural-oral approach* that is usually used depends on the degree and onset of the hearing loss as well as early intervention (Coninx, 1995). Rehabilitation approaches include diagnosis of the hearing impairment, which should be accomplished early—preferably from 0–12 months of life for the neonate—and followed by early intervention through the provision of amplification and development of appropriate educational plans. Early diagnosis and intervention are recommended to take advantage of the plasticity of the CNS, particularly in the first 2 years of life when the central nervous system is considered to be the most sensitive (Coninx, 1995; Downs, 1994). The fitting of hearing aids and, where necessary, the use of cochlear implants, especially by those with profound hearing impairment, can facilitate and enhance development of good communication skills in hearing-impaired individuals without other disabilities. The first step toward successful and effective rehabilitation is assessment. The advent of modern electrophysiologic measures such as auditory brainstem response (ABR) and otoacoustic emissions has improved the accuracy and validity of audiologic assessment of a most difficult and challenging population. Beyond evaluation, standard and scientifically validated aural rehabilitation procedures for people with disabilities are not available (Coninx, 1995). Several reasons have been advanced to explain this situation. Individuals with multiple disabilities are a heterogeneous group. As a result, it is difficult to realistically apply one procedure or approach to all. In addition, people with disabilities constitute a small minority of the general population, and it is not often cost effective to prepare and market products for them on a large scale. As a member of the rehabilitation team, the audiologist needs specific skills to be successful (Table 1.2).

Table 1.2

The Audiologist's Role as a Member of the Rehabilitation Team

The role of the audiologist as a member of an identification team for an individual who is mentally retarded and developmentally disabled includes the following responsibilities:

1. Assessing, describing, and documenting the communicative behaviors and needs of each client and interpreting and integrating the communicative needs with educational and vocational programming.
2. Evaluating various modes of communication with reference to the individual's abilities, disabilities, and communication environment, to develop the most effective means of communication possible, vocal and otherwise.
3. Developing speech and vocal communication to the fullest extent possible, while focusing predominantly on the development of language rather than just speech.
4. Developing intervention procedures and evaluating their effectiveness in producing systems of communication that meet the demands of the environment; interface with other programming; and are appropriate to educational, vocational, and social settings.
5. Incorporating within assessment and intervention program procedures the significant others in the life of the mentally retarded individual including direct caregivers, family members, employers, and other professional team members.
6. Where necessary, training persons to interact with the mentally retarded person who uses an augmentative system of communication.
7. Being a client advocate for audiologic services including diagnostic and rehabilitative services.

American Speech-Language-Hearing Association. (1982). Serving the communicatively handicapped mentally retarded individual. *ASHA, 24*(8), 547–553. (Copyright by the American Speech-Language-Hearing Association. Reprinted with permission.)

PEOPLE WITH OTHER DISABILITIES

Unlike for hearing-impaired people without additional handicaps, for hearing-impaired individuals with other disabilities such as mental retardation, visual impairment, CP, and autism the goals of aural rehabilitation may vary. The extent to which functional residual hearing can be maximized does not depend solely on the degree of the hearing impairment but more so on the extent, degree, or impact of other dominant or multiple existing handicaps that may be present. For individuals with multiple disabilities, such as mental retardation, learning disabilities, and visual impairments, who are also unable to acquire language skills, aural rehabilitation goals need to be modified (Coninx, 1995) for the appropriate levels of development and functioning of the individual. The goal of aural rehabilitation for this group of individuals is not necessarily or primarily the acquisition of spoken language.

Ramsdell (1977) described different levels of hearing from which rehabilitation goals for people with disabilities could be derived. They are as follows: (1) basic level, (2) signal level, (3) symbolic level, and (4) sensomotoric feedback level.

1. *Basic level of hearing.* Hearing is important at this level for the individual to bond with the environment without the feeling of being alone in a silent world. The individual is able to detect environmental sounds; hearing at this level provides a state of awareness about the existence of different kinds of sounds in the environment and their effects.
2. *Signal level of hearing.* The individual is able to recognize and discriminate between various sounds that are important for daily living. For instance, the individual is able to attach meaning to alerting sounds such as fire alarms, sirens, or honks that may signify danger.
3. *Symbolic level of hearing.* This represents the highest level of listening skills in that it involves linguistic processing of abstract sounds and understanding of spoken words.
4. *Sensomotoric feedback level of hearing.* Unlike at the basic, signal, and symbolic levels of hearing, which require receptive skills, at the sensomotoric level, skills are needed to control gross

Table 1.3

Levels of Hearing and Management of People with Disabilities

Levels of hearing	Nature of sounds	Aural rehabilitation goals	Aural rehabilitation methods
Basic	Environmental sounds Traffic noise Music Bell ringing	Reduce individual isolation Facilitate and enhance bonding with the environment Enlarge and enrich the limited world of the deaf-blind Increase the activity level (state of arousal) of passive individuals Create an environment for the individual to experience and enjoy music	Auditory training using environmental sounds, music, and speech Use of hearing aids
Signal	Warning signals Fire alarms Siren Train/car horns	Develop an alerting and warning sound signal system Increase the individual's state of arousal Encourage the use of nonverbal sounds as referential objects	Auditory training using audiovisuals (where necessary) to show source of warning/danger alerting signals
Symbolic	Meaning of words	Stimulate, encourage, and reinforce voicing for demands/requests	Use of hearing aids Speech reading
Sensomotoric	Conversation Speech production	Reduce and discourage unwanted and socially unacceptable voicing	Use of hearing aids Speech reading Story telling
Feedback	Receptive speech Expressive speech	Facilitate cognitive development through various learning tasks	

Adapted from Coninx, F. (1995). Aural rehabilitation issues with multiply handicapped hearing-impaired children. *Scandinavian Audiology Supplement, 41,* 61–65; and Ramsdell, D. (1977). The psychology of the hard of hearing and deafened adult. In Silverman, D. H. (Ed.), *Hearing and deafness.* New York: Holt.

and fine motor activities and to manage speech production for phonation and articulation (Coninx, 1995). For people with severe disabilities aural rehabilitation at the symbolic level is difficult to achieve, because it requires receptive and expressive speech and language skills. However, as Coninx (1995) suggested, attempts to achieve this level should not be neglected or ignored. Instead, there should be individualized goals to reflect the individual's level of development and degree and impact of disability. Some examples of goals derived at different levels of hearing are displayed in Table 1.3.

REFERENCES

American Psychiatric Association. (1994). *Diagnostic and statistical manual of mental disorders* (4th ed.). Washington, DC: American Psychiatric Association.

Ballachanda, B. (2001). Audiological assessment of linguistically and culturally diverse populations. *Audiology Today, 13*(4), 34–35.

Bankaitis, A. E., & Keith, R. W. (1995). Audiological changes associated with HIV infection. *ENT Journal, 75*(5), 353–359.

Batshaw, M. L., & Shapiro, B. K. (1997). Mental retardation. In Batshaw, M. L. (Ed.). *Children with disabilities* (4th ed.). Baltimore: Paul H. Brookes.

Bishop, V. E. (1991). Preschool visually impaired children: A demographic study. *Journal of Visual Impairment and Blindness, 85,* 69–74.

Buncic, J. R. (1987). The blind infant. *Pediatric Clinics of North America, 34,* 1403–1414.

Cherow, E. (Ed.). (1985). *Hearing-impaired children and youth with developmental disabilities.* Washington, DC: Gallaudet College Press.

Coninx, F. (1995). Aural rehabilitation issues with multiply handicapped hearing-impaired children. *Scandinavian Audiology Supplement, 41,* 61–65.

Danseco, E. (1997). Parental beliefs on childhood disability: Insights on culture, child development and intervention. *International Journal of Disability, Development and Education, 44,* 41–52.

Developmental Disabilities Assistance and Bill of Rights Act of 1990, Title 42, U.S.C. 6000–6083. *U.S. Statutes at Large, 104,* 1191–1204.

Downs, M. P. (1994). The case for detection and intervention for infants with hearing impairment. *Seminars in Hearing, 15,* 76–84.

Friedrich, B. W. (1985). The state of the art in audiologic evaluation and management. In Cherow, E. (Ed.). *Children and Youth with Developmental Disabilities.* Washington, DC: Gallaudet College Press.

Grimaldi, L. M., Luzi, L., Martino, G. V., Furlan, R., Nemni, R., Antonelli, A., et al. (1993). Bilateral eighth cranial nerve neuropathy in human immunodeficiency virus infection. *Journal of Neurology, 240*(6), 363–366.

Lalwani, A. K., & Sooy, C. D. (1992). Otologic manifestations of acquired immunodeficiency syndrome. *The Otololaryngological Clinics of North America, 25*(6), 1183–1198.

MCW Health Link. (2002). *Health care for adults with Down syndrome.* Retrieved from http//healthlink.mcw.edu/article/1001820316.html.

Menacker, S. J., & Batshaw, M. L. (1997). Vision: Our window to the world. In Batshaw, M. L. (Ed.). *Children with disabilities* (4th ed.). Baltimore: Paul H. Brookes.

Mardiros, M. (1989). Conception of childhood disability among Mexican-American parents, *Medical Anthropology, 12*, 55–68.

Moazzez, A. H., & Alvi, A. (1998). Head and neck manifestations of AIDS in adults. *American Family Physician, 57*(8), 1813–1822.

Oyiborhoro, J. M. A. (1984). The concept of special education and implications for teacher education in Nigeria. *International Education Journal, 14*(1), 38–43.

Pappas, D. G., Jr., Roland, J. T., Jr., Lim, J., Lai, A., & Hillman, D. E. (1995). Ultrastructural findings in the vestibular end-organs of AIDS cases. *American Journal of Otology, 16*, 140–145.

Ramsdell, D. (1977). The psychology of the hard of hearing and deafened adult. In Silverman, D. H. (Ed.). *Hearing and deafness.* New York: Holt.

Rarey, K. E. (1990). Otologic pathophysiology in patients with human immuno-deficiency virus. *American Journal of Otolaryngology, 11*, 366–369.

Real, R., Thomas, M., & Gerwins, J. M. (1987). Sudden hearing loss and acquired immunodeficiency syndrome. *Otolaryngology Head and Neck Surgery, 97*, 409–412.

Roizen, N. J., Wolters, C., Nicol, T., & Blondis, T. A. (1993). Hearing loss in children with Down syndrome. *Journal of Pediatrics, 123,* S9–S12.

Schaefer, G. B. (1995). Ten syndromes most commonly associated with hearing impairment. *Advances in the genetics of deafness: A Bulletin of the HHIRR, 2*(1).

Soucek, S. & Michaels, L. (1996). The ear in the acquired immunodeficiency syndrome: II. Clinical and audiologic investigation. *American Journal of Otology, 17*(1), 35–39.

Timon, C. I. & Walsh, M. A. (1989). Sudden hearing loss as a presentation of HIV infection. *Journal of Laryngology and Otology; 103,* 1071–1072.

U. S. Census Bureau. (2000). *Coming to America: A profile of the nation's foreign born.* Census brief. Washington, DC: U.S. Government Printing Office.

Voutilainen, R., Jauhiainen, T., & Linkola, H. (1988). Associated handicaps in children with hearing loss. *Scandinavian Audiology Supplement, 30*, 57–59.

Wilson, W. R. (1986). The relationship of the herpes virus family to sudden hearing loss: A prospective clinical study and literature review. *Laryngoscope, 96*, 870–877.

World Health Organization. (1980). International classification of impairments, disabilities, and handicaps: *A manual of classification relating to the consequences of disease.* Geneva: Author.

Worthington, D. W., & Peters, J. F. (1980). Quantifiable hearing and no ABR: Paradox or error? *Ear and Hearing, 1,* 281–285.

SELECTED READINGS

Battle, D. E. (1993). *Communication disorders in multicultural populations.* Boston: Andover Medical Publishers.

Bergman, B., & Rosenhall, U. (2001). Vision and hearing in old age. *Scandinavian Audiology, 30,* 255–263.

Davis, A., Fortnum, H., & Bamford, J. M. (1998). Epidemiologic issues associated with newborn hearing screening. In Bess, F. H. (Ed.). *Children with hearing impairment* (pp. 1–10). Nashville: Vanderbilt Bill Wilkerson Center Press.

Gherman, C. R., Ward, R. R., & Bassis, M. L. (1988). *Pneumocystis carinii* otitis media and mastoiditis as the initial manifestation of the acquired immunodeficiency syndrome. *American Journal of Medicine, 85,* 250–252.

Hirch, A. (1988). Hearing loss and associated handicaps in preschool children. *Scandinavian Audiology Supplement, 30,* 61–64.

Karchmer, M. A. (1985). A demographic perspective. In Cherow, E. (Ed), *Hearing-impaired children and youth with developmental disabilities* (pp. 36–56). Washington, DC: Gallaudet College Press.

Kayser, H. (1998). Outcomes measurement in culturally and linguistically diverse populations. In Frattali, C. M. (Ed). *Measuring outcomes in speech-language pathology* (pp. 225–241). New York: Thieme.

Kramer, L. C., Sullivan, R. F., & Hirsch, L. M. (1979). *Audiological evaluation and aural rehabilitation of the deaf-blind adult.* New York: Helen Keller National Center for Deaf-Blind Youths and Adults.

Mallory, B. L., Charlton, J. I., Nicholls, R. W., & Marfo, K. (1993). Traditional and changing views of disability in developing societies: Causes, consequences, and cautions. *The International Exchange of Experts and Information in Rehabilitation Monograph 53.* Durham, NH: International Exchange of Experts and Information in Rehabilitation.

Mencher, G. T., & Gerber, S. E. (Eds.). (1983). *The multiply handicapped hearing impaired child.* New York: Grune & Stratton.

Mutua, N. K. (2001). Importance of parent's expectations and beliefs in the educational participation of children with mental retardation in Kenya. *Education and Training in Mental Retardation and Developmental Disabilities, 36,* 148–159.

U.S. Census Bureau. (2000a). Table 5: Language spoken at home for the foreign-born population 5 years and over: 1980–1990. Washington, DC: U.S. Government Printing Office.

U.S. Department of Education, Office of Educational Research and Improvement (2000). *Digest of education statistics* (p. 65). Washington, DC: Author.

U.S. Department of Justice. (1991). *Americans with Disabilities Act handbook.* Washington, DC: U.S. Government Printing Office.

Weinstein, B., & Amstel, L. (1986). Hearing loss and senile dementia in the institutionalized elderly. *Clinical Gerontologist, 4*(3), 3–15.

World Health Organization. (1998). ICIDH-2 Beta 1 Field Trials. Retrieved from http://www.who.org.

Audiologic Rehabilitation for People with Disabilities

Assessment and Management

CHAPTER 2

Cerebral Palsy/Developmental Disabilities

John M.A. Oyiborhoro, Ed.D., F.A.A.A., CCC-A
Boro Audiology Clinic
Brooklyn, NY
and
National Institute for People with Disabilities
New York, NY

Cerebral palsy (CP) is not a disease; rather it represents a symptom complex and is an umbrella term used to encompass a group of nonprogressive but often changing disorders of motor function resulting from brain injury or malformation (Kuban & Leviton, 1994; Mutch et al., 1992). Brain lesions that cause various disorders may also contribute to other problems including, but not limited to, mental retardation, seizures, speech and language disorders, and vision and hearing disorders, which are often associated with CP. These other handicaps are also called *developmental disabilities*. They may be severe or chronic and may occur in an individual at 5 years of age or older but must be manifested before the individual attains the age of 22 to qualify as developmental disabilities (Developmental Disabilities Assistance and Bill of Rights Act, 1990). Our definition of CP (especially the causes that are also related to those of the other disabilities) deserves clarification because CP serves as our main disability, along with which other handicaps will be grouped together later.

Many cases of CP result from several types of pre-, peri-, and postnatal events (Evenhuis, 1996; Molnar, 1985; Nelson & Ellenberg, 1978; Pharoah, 1989). Prenatal events, for instance, may be due to maternal infection (such as rubella, cytomegalovirus, toxoplasmosis, herpes, and syphilis), drug and alcohol use during pregnancy, maternal disease, placental insufficiency, and severe circulatory and cardiovascular problems. Perinatal injuries occur during birth and may result from prolonged labor, umbilical cord compression (which often causes anoxia), and head trauma. Postnatal events, on the other hand, occur after birth and may include, but are not limited to, infections such as meningitis, head injuries sustained from accidental childhood falls, cerebrovascular accidents, and blood diseases. However, CP does not include motor disorders resulting from head injuries or cerebrovascular accidents that occur much later in life.

CP is classified according to the parts of the body affected. For instance, in monoplegia, only one limb is affected on one side of the body; in diplegia, legs are mostly affected with a mild muscle tone in the upper body; and in hemiplegia, one side of the body is affected with the arm being more affected than the legs, trunk, or face. The arm is generally bent at the hand, wrist, or elbow with an associated loss of sensation in about 50% of patients (Nelson & Ellenberg, 1978; Pharoah, 1989). In quadriplegia, all four limbs, that is, arms and legs, as well as the trunk are involved. CP may also be classified according to the location of the brain lesion. For example, in spastic (pyramidal) CP, the condition is due to damage to the cerebrum, which controls the initiation and coordination of voluntary body movements (Kuban and Leviton, 1994). If the cerebrum is injured, the integrity of the pyramidal tracts is compromised. The pyramidal tracts unite the motor cortex with efferent nerve fibers that relay motor signals to the muscles to control voluntary movement of body parts. Spastic CP is considered to be the most common type of CP. It is characterized by very limited movement and stiffness. Choreoathetoid (extrapyramidal) CP is another type, which is also referred to as *athetosis*. This condition results from damage to the cerebellum or basal ganglia, which causes abnormal movements of body parts. Thus athetosis is characterized by involuntary and purposeless movement of the head, arms, fingers, legs, and trunk, as well as communication problems. Ataxia is also another condition that is due to an insult to the cerebellum, and it is characterized by an unsteady gait and uncoordinated and shaky movement. If more than one condition occurs in the same individual, such as quadriplegia in an individual with spastic athetosis, it is called mixed CP (Molnar, 1985).

The incidence of moderate to severe cases of CP is estimated to be between 1.5 and 2.5 per 1000 live births (Kuban & Levton, 1994). The estimated prevalence of developmental disabilities ranges from 1 to 2% (American Speech-Language and Hearing Association, 1989). On the other hand, the prevalence of hearing-impaired children with CP or other developmental disabilities may vary widely. Reported estimates range from 5 to 59% (Fisch, 1957; Gersh, 1991; Lloyd & Moore, 1972; Nakano, 1966; Oyiborhoro, 1993; Pruszewicz et al., 1977). Subject selection, subject age, and the definition of what constitutes a hearing loss may in part explain the wide variability in the prevalence of hearing impairment in individuals with CP or developmental disabilities (Levine, 1971; Lloyd & Moore, 1972). With subject selection, for instance, studies indicate that individuals with Down's syndrome have a hearing loss prevalence two to four times greater than that for others with other types of disabilities (Dahle & McCollister, 1986). Generally, the lower the criterion for what constitutes a hearing loss and the lower the cognitive level and functioning of the individual, the greater the prevalence of hearing impairment among people with disabilities (Ray, 2002; Van Schrojenstein Lantman-DeValk et al., 1994). As previously noted, many individuals with CP also have other associated disabilities. Hur (1997) reports that about 40–60% of children with CP have an intellectual disability, 50% have seizure disorders, and 20–60% have visual defects, perceptual dysfunction, communication disorders, behavior problems, social maladjustment, and hearing deficits. It is well known that many of the causes of CP, mental retardation, and other developmental disabilities, such as anoxia, meningitis, cytomegalovirus infection, rubella, and toxoplasmosis, have been associated with hearing impairment as well (Bess & Humes, 1990; Evenhuis, 1996). Some individuals with CP have normal or near-normal cognition and do not have other developmental disabilities. There is also another group of individuals with severe and mixed CP, who have associated disabilities (with varying degrees of severity) that interfere with activities of everyday living.

Both groups are referred to as consumers. The term *consumer* as used here means individuals with CP and/or developmental disabilities. Use of this term removes the negative connotation often associated with disabilities such as CP, mental retardation, Down's syndrome, and autism as well as others. The term is used interchangeably to refer to either people with CP or developmental disabilities or both as necessary. Because CP is not a disease, several techniques have been used to (re)habilitate this population. These methods include the use of surgery to correct some of the physical deformities and the use of prostheses, drugs, physical therapy, speech therapy, and audiologic rehabilitation to ameliorate the challenges presented by CP itself as well as other associated handicapping conditions.

Audiologic evaluation of the physically challenged consumer is particularly challenging. Too often, a lack of response to acoustic signals is misinterpreted to mean a hearing loss, even when a hearing loss is not present (Sigenenthler, 1987). In the population with Down's syndrome peripheral hearing impairment is not only more prevalent, but these consumers also have difficulty storing and retrieving processed information (Swif & Rosin, 1988). The standard behavioral audiologic test battery composed of pure tone and speech audiometry requires that the individual must respond either verbally (e.g., saying "yes") or by the "raising" of a hand when the presented sound signal is heard or by correctly pointing to identify a picture. These response tasks are not suitable for the non-verbal, severely physically challenged consumer with CP because of their limited neuromuscular and cognitive abilities. Unfortunately, audiologic assessment techniques and guidelines for this population are limited. The use of electrophysiologic measures has been strongly suggested by some researchers and clinicians. However, despite the introduction of these objective measures in recent years, conventional behavioral audiometry continues to be widely used among audiologists in the challenging evaluation of consumers with CP. Although electrophysiologic measures such as auditory brainstem response (ABR), otoacoustic emissions (OAE), and immittance can demonstrate the integrity of the auditory structures and pathways, only behavioral measures can reveal their actual functional utility in communication. Furthermore, ABR, which has been an accepted practice for more than 2 decades, has pitfalls, with reported instances of misdiagnosis (Worthington & Peters, 1980). As the reliability of some of the results from ABR—particularly for special populations—come to question, behavioral measures have continued to serve as simple, efficient, cost-effective, and essential clinical tools in hearing evaluation of consumers (Cornacchia et al., 1982; Diefendorf, 2002; Lancioni & Coninx, 1989).

Over the years, clinicians have been compelled to improvise or adapt the traditional audiologic test battery for the evaluation of severely physically challenged consumers. For some consumers, important basic behavioral test components such as speech audiometry have often been ignored. Because people do not communicate in pure tones, it is important to examine other ways, for instance, of assessing speech reception abilities especially of nonverbal, physically challenged consumers. In addition, because of the heterogeneity of the population, standard and uniform evaluation methods are difficult to establish. In the absence of established methods, some clinicians have used word identification by appropriate pointing to the correct pictorial representation. The use of this point-to-response mode, although sometimes suitable for assessing "normal" individuals, is probably unrealistic for evaluation of severely handicapped consumers. We will return to this subject later in the speech audiometry section of this chapter.

In this chapter materials and methods used in the assessment and management of severely physically challenged, hearing-impaired consumers (with CP and/or developmental disabilities) are examined.

Professional encounters with consumers demand that the clinician should possess some specific skills as shown in Table 2.1.

AUDIOLOGIC EVALUATION

BACKGROUND/CASE HISTORY

The first step in audiologic evaluation of a person with disabilities is the taking of a complete case history. The case history is both critical and useful in many respects. First, the process creates the initial opportunity for the clinician to interact directly and closely with the consumer and the family member or the significant other accompanying the individual for the evaluation. Second, a rapport with the consumer and the significant other is established more easily and may prove useful during the actual evaluation. Third, it enables the clinician to form a mental hypothesis about the nature and possible extent of the problem. Fourth, the clinician is able to gain a better insight into the status of the consumer's general health and mental well-being. Fifth, the knowledge gained helps in the choice of appropriate test batteries and protocols to enable the evaluation to be conducted more efficiently and effectively. Choice of the wrong protocols may be attributed to incomplete or inadequate case history taking. This may lead to misdiagnosis and wrong or inappropriate management. Case history taking should encompass the following areas: audiologic background check, communication skills, and medical background (see Appendix at end of this chapter).

Audiologic Background Check

Determining development levels of the consumer is necessary and knowing the consumer's chronologic and mental ages is essential in the choice of methods of testing, test protocols, and interpretation of audiologic findings after evaluation has been completed. Assessment of a 30-year-old consumer who has a mental age of a toddler warrants use of age-appropriate test methods and interpretation of audiologic outcomes.

Sometimes the consumer's legal name on paper may be different from the name he or she is called at home, and the individual may

Table 2.1

Knowledge Areas/Skills an Audiologist Must Possess When Working with Mentally Retarded/Developmentally Disabled Individuals

To meet the standards established by the Code of Ethics, the speech-language pathologist and the audiologist who provide communication services to mentally retarded individuals should possess the following:

1. Knowledge concerning mentally retarded individuals, including information about
   a. factors that contribute to communicative disorders and method of prevention,
   b. preverbal development,
   c. augmentative communication systems,
   d. prognosis, and
   e. therapeutic techniques.
2. The ability to deal with a variety of handicapping conditions (i.e., aberrant behavior, seizures, feeding problems, etc.) that are evidenced by mentally retarded individuals in addition to the communication disorder.
3. Expertise in ongoing diagnosis and assessment (through formal and informal, standardized and nonstandardized procedures) of the type, nature, and severity of the communication disorder evidenced by a mentally retarded person.
4. The knowledge required to plan and implement an intervention program that will allow the mentally retarded individual to develop communication skills, vocal or otherwise, that are appropriate to the individual's living environment and potential.
5. Skill in cooperating in an interdisciplinary team approach to provide services in the clinical, educational, or living milieu of the retarded person.
6. The ability to educate colleagues, administrators, parents, direct care staff, and the community about mentally retarded individuals and their communication needs. This includes the ability to conduct staff training, establish home programs, and involve paraprofessionals to meet the needs of mentally retarded individuals.
7. Insight into knowledge and techniques of other professions that deal with mentally retarded people.

American Speech-Language-Hearing Association (1982). Serving the communicatively handicapped mentally retarded individual. *ASHA, 24,* 547–553. (Copyright by the American Speech-Language-Hearing Association. Reprinted with permission.)

become unresponsive when the legal name is called. If the consumer is more used to his or her nickname, it is usually better to use this preferred name. Use of the preferred name tends to facilitate bonding and to create a good rapport with the consumer.

To obtain information about the hearing status of the consumer, parents should be asked the following questions: Is there any history of hearing loss in your family? Do you suspect that your child has a hearing loss? Has your child ever used a hearing aid before? The clinician should be aware that all answers may be negative, because parents of children with CP and other disabilities may not be prepared to receive more bad news about an additional disability they have to cope with if this is the first audiologic appointment or an appointment to obtain a second opinion on the hearing status of their child. If, for instance, a parent suspects the presence of a hearing loss, he or she may be more receptive and cooperative during counseling. A possible "honest" answer helps the clinician in forming a mental hypothesis about what is going on auditorily and narrowing the choice of the test battery to be used. If a parent says that there is no history of hearing loss in the family or that the child is not suspected of having a hearing problem, but he or she states that the child was wearing hearing aids until they were lost a few months ago, this inconsistency signals a red flag for the clinician. Probing further about the type of hearing aid, length of time the device was used before being lost, and results of previous evaluations may provide a better understanding about the nature and extent of hearing loss.

Communication Skills

The clinician needs to know the predominant language that the consumer is exposed to at home or at the residence, if the consumer is institutionalized. Many consumers can receive a misdiagnosis because of a language barrier. If the consumer does not understand the necessary test instructions clearly before an evaluation, it is likely that appropriate and expected responses may not be obtained. In this case, there is a need to provide an interpreter for the consumer's native language to be certain that test instructions are properly understood and also to help address issues arising from previous evaluations. If, for example, a consumer's primary or predominant language at home is Spanish or Russian, it would be more appropriate to use this language to give test instructions and to provide audiologic counseling after the test is completed.

Do younger consumers recognize the voices of their parents? Or can older consumers differentiate the voices of their close caregivers or support staff? What are their reactions to loud sounds? People with autism are known to have unusual auditory deficits (Konstantareas & Homatidis, 1987; Schlopler, Reichler, DeVellis, & Daly, 1980). Autistic consumers often show inconsistent responses to acoustic stimuli. They are usually unresponsive to human voices and often avoid making any direct eye contact. Consumers with autistic features are hypersensitive to sounds (McCormick, 1995) and may make quick responses to loud "nonsense" or mechanical sounds, especially if such sounds are presented when the consumer is in a calm and undistracted state.

Does the consumer respond to his or her name if the caller is out of visual field? Does the consumer respond or is the consumer able to identify a conventional telephone ring, doorbell, or smoke alarm? Has the consumer worn an amplification device before? If the answer is yes, was the consumer satisfied with the device(s)? Many consumers reject hearing devices because of overfitting. Overfitting may originate from inappropriate selection of devices based on flawed test results. One additional question is: Can the consumer verbalize any words or obey commands? The answers to these questions may give an insight into the presence, nature, and extent of a hearing impairment.

Medical Background

Information about specific medical conditions is obtained at this time. Questions to ask include the following. Are there any obvious craniofacial anomalies? What specific disabilities or syndromes are present? Refer to the list of top 10 syndromes associated with hearing impairment in Chapter 1. Do some of these syndromes have an impact on the auditory system? Were there any maternal diseases or pre-, peri-, or postnatal events during the consumer's birth? If there was a period of hospitalization, what was the length of hospital stay and the type of medication taken by the consumer (or the mother during or after delivery)? Were any of the drugs used known to be ototoxic? The mental age of the person is important in selecting the test battery components and in choosing the test protocols. For instance, a

30-year-old adult with a mental age of a 2-year-old obviously needs a test mode and interpretation different from those used for a normal 30-year-old adult. Does the individual have a history of ear infection? If hearing loss is present from a previous evaluation, what type of hearing loss was present? Does the consumer have limited visual acuity? The extent of the consumer's vision limitation will dictate how much modification should be made if visual reinforcement audiometry (VRA) has been selected as a technique to use during evaluation. A good case history of the consumer provides an invaluable initial step in the choice of appropriate test batteries and test protocols before evaluation. With a knowledge of the dominant disability (or associated disabilities), mental age, and communication and motor skills, the clinician is able to form a mental hypothesis of the degree, type, and configuration of the hearing loss. The clinician should have an idea about the final outcome of the evaluation based on the case history before proceeding.

Other Consumer Information

Ask the person who accompanied the consumer for information about the nature of their relationship. That is, is the person a direct caregiver or blood relation? This information will determine the kinds of questions the clinician should ask to take into consideration the sensitivities of and/or perceptions of the accompanying person, especially if he or she is the consumer's parent. Creating a good rapport with the accompanying parents or direct caregivers is almost as important as creating and maintaining a good rapport with the consumer for four reasons: (1) they can become the clinician's friend and partner in the evaluation process, (2) they can provide more detailed information about the consumer's likes and dislikes that are likely to interfere with or compromise test results but that are not usually adequately recorded in the consumer's chart; (3) maintaining their presence can reassure the consumer that he or she is in safe and familiar territory because there is someone familiar who can calm fears; and (4) they can provide information about the types of medications the consumer is taking and dosages. Accompanying persons can also provide information as to whether the consumer is in a happy, sad, angry, or sick (worse than usual) mode. This information alone can help the clinician decide whether to suspend or cancel the session or determine how to cope with the consumer's emotional mode.

OTOSCOPY

After history taking, the next step in the evaluation process is otoscopic examination. This involves a visual inspection of the ear and ear canal. With the advent of video otoscopy, this procedure has become more exciting and fun for the consumer, accompanying caregiver or parent, and the clinician. First, the pinna and external auditory canals are examined for any structural abnormalities that may reveal features of syndromes known to be associated with hearing impairment. Abnormally small or missing pinna and stenotic or missing external auditory canals are some of the structural ear defects associated with syndromes such as Down's, Treacher Collin, and Alport's. These syndromes are associated with a high incidence of hearing impairment. The clinician should check for impacted or excessive cerumen accumulation in the ear canal, which is a frequent and chronic problem in this population (Crandell & Roeser, 1993; Evenhuis, 1995) and a common cause of conductive hearing loss. The incidence of impacted/excessive cerumen in this population is much higher than that in the general population (Evenhuis, 1995). Ray (2002) provided three reasons for this occurrence:

1. Consumers tend to have anatomic ear differences such as the stenotic (narrowing) ear canals seen in Down's syndromes, which tend to facilitate cerumen accumulation.
2. Physiologic differences on how cerumen is produced among consumers and the general population coupled with poor hygiene.
3. Inability of the consumer (because of cognitive deficits) to complain about ear discomfort and hearing loss resulting from impacted cerumen.

An additional reason that might be added is the lack of annual or periodic audiologic services to help maintain better hearing health for these consumers. Thus periodic audiologic evaluations should be recommended for these consumers and appropriate referrals made for cerumen management.

The ear canal is further examined for canal drainage and integrity of the tympanic membrane. Video otoscopy makes this visualization easier, and the consumer is often exited about seeing "inside the ear," which may create more interest in subsequent procedures. With video otoscopy, both the consumer and the accompanying caregiver or family member can visualize the ear canal together to exclude excessive cerumen accumulation or the presence of a foreign body. Some consumers do not want their ears touched and may vigorously resist otoscopic examination. It is not advisable for the clinician to push too far, because the consumer's resistance may be hardened by such action, thereby discouraging further participation in subsequent procedures. Although immittance measurements should normally follow otoscopy, we will discuss these later in the physiologic testing section. Otherwise, it is good to check the status of the middle ear immediately after otoscopy. However, some consumers, particularly children, resist the use of the probe tip as in immittance measurements. Again, it is not advisable to force the issue, but rather to return to the procedure after speech audiometry has been completed.

PURE TONE AUDIOMETRY

Some consumers with CP or other disabilities, who have mild disabilities or near-normal developmental conditions, do not present many difficulties in testing. Such consumers can be evaluated using the conventional methods that are applicable to the general population. The audiometric findings for consumers with CP in particular may show some similarities in terms of configuration and symmetry of hearing impairment, mostly in the high-frequency range (Mysak, 1971; Ray, 2002). In pure tone audiometry, the objective always is to use conventional methods and protocols to obtain accurate hearing thresholds. Although this is possible for consumers with mild disabilities or near-normal developmental conditions, it is not a realistic goal for consumers who are nonverbal or who have severe to profound neurologic, physical, motor, and cognitive deficits. The primary and realistic goal in this group of consumers, therefore, is to rule out bilateral moderate to profound hearing loss, especially in the speech frequencies of 500–2000 Hz (Gans & Gans, 1993; Siegenthaler, 1987).

Involuntary body movements are very common in the CP population with spastic athetosis. If these movements become vigorous and prolonged, they may interfere with testing. Such rhythmic, vigorous body movements may create masking noise in the 30–40 dB range (Mysak, 1971), which may compromise test result accuracy. Furthermore, concentration and responses to the primary auditory pure tone signals being presented become difficult for the consumer to attend to.

CONVENTIONAL PURE TONE AUDIOMETRY

For consumers with higher cognitive levels who do not have serious additional disabilities, conventional pure tone audiometry can be performed. This procedure involves presenting pure tone signals and having the consumer respond whenever the signal is heard by saying "yes," raising a hand, or pushing a button. Our preference is to ask consumers to say "yes" each time the signal is heard because this keeps them more alert and focused on the task. Some consumers prefer to describe the loudness or softness of the tones, which is also acceptable. The use of insert earphones is encouraged and advocated. Figure 2.1 shows a consumer being prepared by a clinician for an evaluation using insert earphones.

Insert earphones are disposable and can help in maintaining good hygiene and infection control because a new pair is used for each consumer. For consumers whose neck region is so spastic that the head rests permanently on one shoulder or so hypotonic that the head hardly maintains a supine position, insert earphones best serve our evaluation needs. If the head of the consumer is too small, as seen in microcephalus and sometimes in Down's syndrome, or too big, as in hydrocephalus, or if the pinnae are malformed, the use of earphones may not be possible because they may not fit properly. If the earphones are too large, they may cause an overlapping of the ears, which allows some of the sound stimulus to leak out. In hydrocephalic consumers with large heads, it is always difficult to adjust the headphones to sufficiently cover the ears, and this may also cause sound leakage from the standard earphone. If insert earphones are used efficiently, they can lessen problems with collapsible ear canals and problems with sound leakage and minimize the increased interaural attenuation seen with standard earphones (Wilber, 2002). The presence of

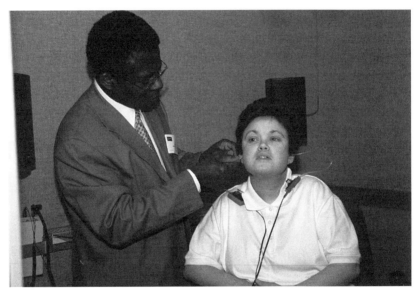

Figure 2.1   A clinician prepares a consumer for an evaluation using insert earphones. (Photo printed with permission.)

collapsible ear canals is suspected if immittance measurements findings are normal, but a high-frequency conductive hearing loss is present (Kile, 1996). In general, we can state five good reasons why the use of insert earphones is recommended:

1. They are comfortable and lightweight.
2. There is no need for masking because of the increased interaural attenuation, which is minimized.
3. The chance for ear canal collapse is minimal.
4. They are disposable and hygienic.
5. Sound is delivered closer to the tympanic membrane compared with conventional earphones.

With consumers who have high levels of cognitive function, it is still important to state and restate test instructions before and during the evaluation. Restating the instructions periodically helps to keep the consumer focused and gives the clinician the assurance that the consumer is engaged with the ongoing evaluation. For consumers who are nonverbal or who have severe neurologic problems or cognitive deficits or who are uncooperative, other test methods and response modes should be used.

Behavioral Observation Audiometry

Behavioral observation audiometry (BOA) is a test method that assesses the general behavioral changes of a consumer to sounds. BOA has been used as an audiologic procedure mostly for infants with mental ages younger than 6 months. However, this technique can also be used for nonverbal consumers with severe cognitive and neuromotor deficits. BOA can serve as a screening tool (Thompson & Weber, 1974) or as an evaluation tool (Talbott, 1987). In BOA the clinician is usually the examiner and other support staff, who are trained to act as judges for observing any behavioral changes or responses whenever auditory stimuli are presented, are also involved. The clinician alerts the judges in the test room before the presentation of auditory signals. The judges and the clinician will then determine whether a response was indeed an actual response or not a response. Test stimuli that are presented through insert earphones or loudspeakers may be warble tone, narrow band noise, or a live voice. Because pure tones and warble tone are much more difficult to attend to, it is preferable to use narrow band noise signals with this population. The use of narrow band noise signals can yield valid and reliable hearing thresholds even better than use of pure tones (Sanders & Josey, 1970). In real life people do not listen to pure tones, and it is much easier for them to attend to narrow band noise signals. The draw-back with the use of narrow band noise signals is that they tend to underestimate hearing thresholds in the higher frequencies; however, they still retain the value of frequency specificity like pure tones (Sanders & Josey, 1970). Consumers give a wide variety of responses. Because many consumers' responses are prone to habituation, it is impor-tant for both the judges and the clinician to be vigilant to the initial response to signals that were presented. Once a consumer's response to an initial signal has become habituated, a new and novel stimulus will be needed to elicit a new response. If the initial stimulus were to be warble tone, it might be useful to alternate with narrow band noise or live voice. However, to maintain consistency with one stimulus, the alternate signals merely serve as distractions or interludes to make the initial stimulus novel and different all over again. Whenever consumers habituate to signals, they lose interest, and it is difficult to evoke responses even at significantly higher intensity levels of presentation. It is important to note consumer's chronologic and mental age of development and also the individual's medical disposition. A knowledge of results of a previous audiogram may bias the outcome of the current evaluation. Thus even if the previous evaluation was done by the same clinician, it is advisable to use it only for the purpose of comparison after the new evaluation has been concluded. As previously noted, consumers display a wide array of behaviors in response to auditory stimuli. These can be grouped into two categories: (1) attentive orienting and (2) reflexive behaviors described by Diefendor (2002) as displayed in Table 2.2. According to Diefendorf (2002), consumers with higher levels of cortical functioning who can attach meaning to sound are more likely to exhibit attentive or orienting types of behaviors to auditory stimuli than are those who present the reflexive type of behavior but who cannot attach much meaning to sound.

A major limitation to the use of BOA that is often cited is that it measures a consumer's responsiveness to sound rather than sensitivity to sound. Despite this limitation, BOA can be used as one portion of a test battery approach for evaluation.

Table 2.2

Behavioral Responses of Children with Severe Disabilities

Behavior Type	Responses
Attentive/orienting	Smiling
	Laughing
	Crying
	Grimacing
	Searching
	Pointing
	Slightly repeatable movement of body parts
Reflexive	Body startle
	Initiation or cessation of sucking
	Increased or decreased sucking, eye blink, or flutter

Adapted from Diefendorf, A. O. (2002). Detection and assessment of hearing loss in infants and children. In J. Katz (Ed.). *Handbook of clinical audiology* (5th ed.). New York: Lippincott Williams and Wilkins.

Visual Reinforcement Audiometry

Visual reinforcement audiometry (VRA) is a method of obtaining hearing thresholds that is most appropriate with severely physically challenged consumers (Decker & Wilson, 1977; Talbott, 1987). VRA is an operant conditioning response and can be used to evaluate consumers aged 1.5–2 years and older (Evenhuis, 1996). During operant conditioning, the auditory stimulus presented evokes the consumer's response, which results in a head-turn toward the direction of the sound (localization). A head-turn toward the direction of the sound becomes the operant behavior that is rewarded by giving positive reinforcement. If the positive reinforcement is of interest and value to the consumer, his or her attention will be sustained and the head-turn will continue whenever the auditory stimulus is presented until the procedure is completed. To obtain valid and reliable results with VRA, training sessions are necessary. The training trials or conditioning involves pairing the auditory stimulus with a reinforcer. For instance, presentation of sound is paired with illumination of a clown or doll above a loudspeaker. Once the clinician is satisfied that desired responses have been achieved consistently upon presentation of auditory stimuli after a few trials, the actual evaluation can then begin. For very young consumers, it is advisable to ask the parent or significant other whether the individual is frightened by loud sounds or moving toys. This information is important so that the consumer is not upset inadvertently. Some reinforcers that provoke laughter, curiosity, and interest in one consumer may evoke the opposite reaction of anger, crying, and lack of interest in another. Thus the conditioning periods should also serve to screen reinforcers that are likely to be problematic during the actual procedure. In VRA, visual reinforcers are mostly three-dimensional objects—usually brightly colored clowns or toys that can move when activated. Young (1994) suggests caution in using VRA with consumers who have a history of seizures that can be triggered by bright or flickering visual stimuli. VRA can be difficult or almost impossible as an evaluation technique for some consumers with CP whose head and neck region is so spastic or so hypotonic that head control is very difficult to maintain (Siegenthaler, 1987). The use of insert earphones with this group of consumers and in those who are microcephalic or hydrocephalic can be very convenient and successful (Widen & O'Grady, 2002). Because consumers can quickly habituate their responses, it is wise to work fast, especially through initial conditioning trial periods. The clinician may talk to, smile at, and interact with the consumer. This creates better bonding of the consumer with the clinician and removes or reduces the expectation of an impending dangerous event that is about to happen in the test environment. The examination should be made as free of tension as possible for the consumer. VRA can be an effective evaluation tool for use with consumers who have severe to profound cognitive deficits (Decker & Wilson, 1977; Talbott, 1987; Thompson, Wilson, & More, 1979).

AIR PUFF AUDIOMETRY

Air puff audiometry is a new procedure (Lancioni & Coninx, 1995) that has been used with consumers who have severe disabilities and multiple handicaps. Air puff audiometry is a classic conditioning procedure in which an air puff (unconditioned stimulus) is paired to an auditory stimulus (conditioned stimulus). The air puff can be directed to the consumer's face, eyes, or neck and evokes defensive responses such as eye blinks or head turns. This procedure is not yet widely used clinically, especially in this country. The air puff is generated from an air cylinder filled with compressed air, and a sound generating system provides the auditory stimulus with which the air puff is paired. Lancioni and Coninx (1995) reported that air puff audiometry is as effective as VRA in the assessment of multiply handicapped consumers.

OTHER BEHAVIORAL EVALUATION TOOLS

Conditioned play audiometry (CPA) and tangible reinforcement operant conditioning audiometry (TROCA) are other behavioral evaluation tools based on operant conditioning techniques. In these two evaluation procedures the consumer must make physical motor responses to auditory stimuli.

Tangible Reinforcement Operant Conditioning Audiometry

In TROCA the consumer is required to push a button, which dispenses a tangible reinforcer (usually something edible such as an M&M or a token). TROCA, unlike other behavioral evaluation methods, was developed using developmentally disabled consumers in the process and has been used by many clinicians in evaluating hearing sensitivities of consumers (Bess & Humes, 1990). A major drawback with TROCA is in the choice of appropriate reinforcers, especially for consumers with severe to profound disabilities (Friedrich, 1985). Even a simple edible reinforcer such as an M&M may be dangerous if, for example, the consumer is allergic to peanuts or other foods. TROCA does not work for many consumers with CP because of their involuntary movements and the presence of primitive reflexes. These physical challenges tend to compound the consumer's inability to make appropriate responses whenever auditory stimuli are presented.

Conditioned Play Audiometry

During CPA, the consumer is conditioned to drop blocks in the bucket or stack up donut rings in response to an auditory stimulus. Evenhuis (1996) suggested the use of CPA with consumers in the developmental age range of between 2.5 to 3 years and older. However, apart from the consumer's level of cognition, the presence or absence of physical challenges should constitute a major consideration. The goal of pure tune audiometry is to obtain the degree, configuration, and type of hearing loss. In our practice we consider 30 dB hearing level (HL) as acceptable for "normal" hearing, giving allowances for the challenges posed by the individual's disability.

SPEECH AUDIOMETRY

Pure tones are used to assess the degree and type of hearing impairment. However, people do not communicate in pure tones. With speech audiometry we are able to assess a consumer's ability to perceive and recognize various speech sounds. Therefore the main goal of speech audiometry is to provide information about the consumer's ability to perceive speech. Because many consumers generally respond faster to more familiar speech sounds than to sounds that are not familiar, speech materials are generally composed of a wide range of frequencies and tend to elicit quicker responses than pure tones (Ray, 2002; Rittmanic, 1971). Sometimes speech audiometry becomes the main behavioral clinical evaluation tool available when pure tone audiometry cannot be performed, but speech audiometry cannot provide definitive information about the type, degree, and configuration of hearing impairment. Mandell (2002) described four response tasks in evaluating speech perception ability:

1. Detection—the ability to determine whether a speech stimulus is present.
2. Discrimination—the ability to distinguish between whether two stimuli are the same or different.
3. Identification—the ability to recognize a stimulus and identify it by repeating it or pointing to a pictorial representation.
4. Comprehension—the ability to decode or understand the meaning of the speech stimulus.

Mandell (2002) suggested the use of various speech stimuli, including a range of phonemes syllables, words, phrases, sentences, and connected discourse, to assess each response task. Assessing these response tasks is more difficult in severely physically challenged consumers, particularly those who are nonverbal and so are unable to repeat, point to, or write words that are presented by the clinician during speech audiometry. For consumers with CP and other disabilities who have normal or near-normal cognitive abilities and whose physical challenges can be described as mild, unmodified speech audiometry can be performed. That is, the consumer's speech recognition threshold (SRT) and word recognition (WR) ability can be assessed just like those of the general population by using and following the standard and usual protocols. However, it is suggested that words which are more familiar and which can evoke some excitement be used.

Speech Recognition Threshold

We suggest the use of words such as ice cream, cupcake, hot dog, baseball, football, playground, wheelchair, airplane, railroad, raincoat, and toothbrush, which are familiar to most consumers. Speech audiometry can provide information about the degree of hearing loss and how the consumer functions auditorily in the low, mid, or high frequencies. In severely physically challenged consumers, the conventional test and response modes must be modified to make the procedure more effective and accurate. Byers and Bristow (1990) suggested the eyegaze response mode for use with these consumers. In the eyegaze response, nonverbal consumers are to turn their heads toward and gaze with their eyes or point to the pictorial representation of the words presented. However, this response depends on the degree of mobility and voluntary control of the head and neck region. In our practice we have modified the use of two-dimensional pictorial representation and replaced it instead with three-dimensional models of words presented. The three-dimensional models of actual objects, in our judgment, are more appealing and exciting and make more sense to a lot of consumers than speech items, especially for those with lower cognitive abilities. Speech audiometry items can be handmade in clinics with actual three-dimensional objects such as an apple, an ice cream cone, a hot dog, or an airplane, which are then placed on clear acrylic boards using Velcro. In some cases, we have used "word command" phrases, when reliable responses could not otherwise be obtained, but phrases such as "head up," "hand down," "close eyes," "open eyes," and "stand up," may require some degree of comprehension for the consumer to perform these tasks.

Speech Awareness Threshold

The speech awareness threshold (SAT) becomes the only alternative if consumers are unable to participate in SRT or word command procedures because of limited cognitive abilities or severe neurologic defects. Although the goal of SRT is to determine the lowest level that can identify speech stimuli correctly, 50% of the time SAT merely determines the lowest level at which an individual can detect the presence of speech 50% of the time. SAT can be conducted using test items that provide frequency-specific information for low-, mid-, and high-frequency specific information such as /a/, /i/, /u/, /sh/, and /s/ (Ling, 1978). Mandell (2002) suggested the use of /ba/ and /bu/ for assessing low-frequency components, /sh/ for mid to high frequencies, and /s/ for assessing mainly high frequencies.

Word Recognition Ability

Generally, regular word recognition test items used for the general population can also be used for consumers who have mild or near-normal cognition. For more developmentally challenged consumers with CP, speech items used with children can be modified and used (Evenhuis, 1996). For instance, the use of modified versions of the Word Intelligibility by Picture Identification (WIPI) word list (Ross & Lerman, 1970) can be used. With the use of Velcro, models of words presented can be placed on acrylic boards similar to those used for SRT. Usually it is easier for consumers to identify words with three-dimensional models because they look more real than two-dimensional pictures or diagrams of objects. Words for familiar items found in the consumer's environment such as spoon, fork, cup, chair, milk, straw, cake, shirt, and pants can be used. In addition, word commands can be useful, especially with non-verbal consumers without serious physical limitations who can comprehend and follow simple word command instructions. Word recognition ability can be measured by the use of phrases such as show me your head, mouth, eyes, nose, lips, teeth, etc. For nonverbal consumers who are more physically compromised, the eyegaze technique previously described under the heading Speech Recognition Threshold can be used.

ELECTROPHYSIOLOGIC MEASURES

Accurate and reliable evaluation findings are essential for selecting appropriate intervention strategies and for achieving desired rehabilitative outcomes. An inability to respond to presented test stimuli because of hypotonia, severe spasticity, severe to profound cognitive deficits, unco-operative behavior, and sometimes unpredictable behaviors of consumers with CP and autistic features who may constantly grab test equipment or move around the test environment during the evaluation, often makes assessment very challenging and difficult to accomplish. Thus physio-logic measures such as ABR, OAE, and immittance have become almost routine methods in hearing assessment.

Immittance Measurements

After otoscopic examination of the ear canals to ensure that the pathway is free of excessive cerumen accumulation, debris, and foreign objects, immittance measurements are taken. Immittance is an important objective evaluation tool used to evaluate the integrity of the middle ear system of consumers, particularly those with Down's syndrome for whom middle ear pathologic conditions are very prevalent. It is often stated that testee cooperation or participation during electrophysiologic measures is not important, unlike with behavioral assessment. However, for consumers who have spastic athetosis and often exhibit involuntary movements, obtaining physiologic measurements including immittance can be a challenge. Obtaining and maintaining air-tight seals to accomplish the immittance procedure can be difficult, especially if the consumer refuses to cooperate by ripping the probe tips from the ears. This is very common with consumers who have behavioral problems. Immittance measurements comprise three main components: tympanometry, static compliance, and acoustic reflex measurements. Immittance measures the mobility of the tympanic membrane, integrity of the ossicles (middle ear bones), Eustachian tube function, middle ear pressure, and the stapedial acoustic reflex. When tympanometric findings are normal, the absence of acoustic reflexes may indicate loss of stapedial muscle function or severe sensorineural hearing loss or dysfunction of the acoustic-facial reflex (Maurizi, Ottaviani, & Paludetti, 1995).

Once the consumer can cooperate, tympanometric and acoustic reflex measurements can be taken. Results from these measurements are similar compared with those for the general population (Fulton & Lamb, 1972). However, in the consumer population with Down's syndrome, in whom conductive hearing loss is very prevalent due to Eustachian tube dysfunction (MCW Health Link, 2002), tympanometric abnormalities range widely from 32 to 68% (Keiser, Montague, Wold, Maune, & Pattison, 1981; Mazzoni, Ackley, & Nash, 1994).

Stenotic ear canals, commonly found in Down's syndrome, can compromise tympanometric measurements, especially when some amount of cerumen is present in the ear canals (Kile, 1996). Therefore external ear canals should be thoroughly inspected before immittance measurements are taken. Acoustic reflex measurements have been used to determine hearing thresholds (Green & Margolis, 1983; Hannley, 1984; Jerger, Burney, Mauldin, & Crump, 1974; Niemeyer & Sesterhenn, 1974) in severely impaired consumers. With the advent of ABR and OAE, the use of this procedure appears to be diminishing.

Otoacoustic Emissions

OAE are a fast, cost-effective, and frequency-specific tool for screening auditory sensitivity in people with disabilities (Evenhuis, 1996). OAE provide information about the integrity of cochlear structure; that is, OAE give us information about outer hair cell function and inner ear micromechanics or hearing in general.

OAE are usually present in ears with hearing thresholds in the range of 30–35 dB HL or better. The presence of OAE indicate normal functioning of outer hair cells. However, this procedure does not provide the degree or configuration of hearing loss.

When hearing loss is present and greater than 30 dB HL, transient OAE are absent. On the other hand, if the hearing loss is greater than 35–40 dB HL, distortion product emission OAE are absent (Hall, 2000).

The presence of middle ear diseases can cause abnormal OAE findings (Hall, 2000; Sutton, Gleadle, & Rowe, 1996) because middle ear pathologic conditions that may cause (conductive hearing loss) limit the intensity of sound reaching the cochlea, which in turn limits the intensity of cochlea response. Furthermore, middle ear pathologic conditions limit the intensity of the echo that is transmitted back to the tympanic membrane from the cochlea, which may or may not be detected as a signal. Thus it is wise to rule out middle ear pathologic conditions before obtaining OAE. Because OAE are frequency specific, they can be absent in regions where hearing is greater than 40 dB HL and present in frequency regions where hearing sensitivity is better than 30 dB HL in the same ear.

Auditory Brainstem Response Testing

ABR is in widespread use as an objective measure of cochlea and retrocochlear pathologic condition. The procedure is noninvasive and is not affected by sleep, sedation, or anesthesia (Hall, 2000; Maurizi et al., 1995). ABR can be used to obtain accurate hearing thresholds, except for hearing losses greater than 80 dB HL in the frequency range of 1000–4000 Hz. Because of these attributes, ABR is often used to evaluate the hearing thresholds of severe to profound mentally retarded consumers who otherwise would be untestable (Benham-Dunster & Dunster, 1985; Smith and Simmons, 1982). However, in some consumers, ABR can be absent even when other test measures show that only a mild hearing loss is present. It has been reported that ABRs may not be detected if the lesion occurs at the brainstem level even with normal cochlear responses (Hall, 2002; Kraus, Ozdamar, Stein, & Reed, 1984; Maurizi, Altissimi, Ottaviani, Paludetti, & Bambini, 1982). Because of the fragile nature of some consumers, the need for sedation and possibility of complications that might result was a source of concern, but many consumers can be tested without the need for sedation (Ray, 2002; Smyth, 1984). However, with consumers who have CP, sedation is often needed (Siegenthaler, 1987), except for those whose conditions are so severe that they are unable to relax their head and neck regions (Ray, 2002). ABR findings are not foolproof. Some ABR results have been found to be at variance with behavioral evaluation outcomes. ABRs may be absent even when there is normal hearing sensitivity (Worthington & Peters, 1980). Additionally, ABR findings can overestimate or underestimate a hearing loss (Gans & Gans, 1993).

Middle Latency Responses

Middle latency responses (MLRs) represent responses from the activation of the auditory pathway between primary cortex and the auditory thalamus, and these responses occur between 15 and 50 msec. Measurement of these responses presents an advantage because they are said to be more detectable near thresholds (Maurizi et al., 1984). There are, however, some practical concerns relating to the influence of maturational effects as well as test parameters, and other variables such as sleep or sedation may have an impact on test outcomes. In general, MLR testing is suggested if ABRs are absent or cannot be obtained.

INTERPRETATION OF TEST OUTCOMES

To obtain more reliable and accurate results, it is best to combine the three main electrophysiologic measures, immittance, OAE, and ABR, with outcomes of behavioral evaluation (Table 2.3). For consumers who have CP and other disabilities and whose hearing is within the normal range and who also have normal middle ear function, aural rehabilitation would be recommended only if communication skills are limited and there is need to facilitate and enhance the development of speech and language skills. Petrak (2000) described four combinations of psysiologic test outcomes as follows.

ABNORMAL ABR, ABSENT OAE, ABSENT ACOUSTIC REFLEXES, NORMAL TYMPANOGRAM

These outcomes typically suggest a possible severe to profound sensorineural hearing impairment. Behavioral audiologic evaluation is suggested to indicate the degree and configuration of hearing loss so that appropriate hearing devices can be selected and fitted. This will also help direct the (re)habilitation and educational options to be chosen.

NORMAL ABR, ABNORMAL OAE, ABNORMAL TYMPANOGRAM, ABSENT ACOUSTIC REFLEX

These findings suggest a possible middle ear pathologic condition. The consumer needs medical follow-up. A repeat of immittance and OAE measures is suggested in 4–6 weeks.

ABNORMAL ABR, NORMAL OAE, NORMAL TYMPANOGRAM

These outcomes suggest possible auditory neuropathy (Don & Kwong, 2002). Consumers typically have some hearing loss, but their word recognition scores are significantly poorer than the degree

Table 2.3

Electrophysiologic Evaluation Outcomes and Management

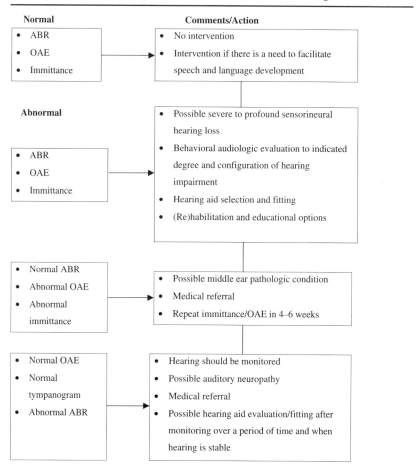

Normal	Comments/Action
• ABR • OAE • Immittance	• No intervention • Intervention if there is a need to facilitate speech and language development

Abnormal

• ABR • OAE • Immittance	• Possible severe to profound sensorineural hearing loss • Behavioral audiologic evaluation to indicated degree and configuration of hearing impairment • Hearing aid selection and fitting • (Re)habilitation and educational options
• Normal ABR • Abnormal OAE • Abnormal immittance	• Possible middle ear pathologic condition • Medical referral • Repeat immittance/OAE in 4–6 weeks
• Normal OAE • Normal tympanogram • Abnormal ABR	• Hearing should be monitored • Possible auditory neuropathy • Medical referral • Possible hearing aid evaluation/fitting after monitoring over a period of time and when hearing is stable

Adapted after Petrak, M. R. (2000, August). Integrating physiologic technologies for hearing evaluation in infants and small children: An overview. Unpublished handout: ICS Medical.

of hearing loss would indicate. Consumers' hearing should be monitored over time to see if changes might occur or hearing is stable.

MANAGEMENT

Parents or significant others of consumers with hearing impairment usually receive audiologic counseling. The degree, type, and configuration of the hearing loss as well as its impact on speech and language development are explained in simple and nontechnical terms. If there is evidence of a genetic component to the hearing loss from case history information, then a referral for genetic counseling is warranted. Generally, behind-the-ear (BTE) hearing instruments are recommended for children. The likelihood of losing a BTE hearing aid that is attached to an earmold would be less than that of losing a much smaller in-the-ear (ITE) hearing aid. In addition, only the earmold in BTE hearing aids would require changing periodically as the child grows. The cost of obtaining a replacement earmold is much less than that of rebuilding or recasing an ITE hearing aid. Body hearing aids are not very popular anymore because the power output of many BTE hearing aids is now comparable to that of body aids. To reduce the chances of losing a hearing aid, otoclips can be used to attach the device to the consumer's clothing. The user's name can be written on the hearing device, especially if the consumer lives in an institution, to avoid the risk of the device being mixed up with those of other users. Mix-ups are common with ITE hearing instruments that look very much alike.

The accuracy and effectiveness of selecting and fitting hearing devices have been revolutionized with the introduction of programmable digital hearing aids and speech mapping. With speech mapping, a consumer's benefit from a hearing instrument can be measured and known before the devices are dispensed. Although more expensive than analog hearing aids, digital hearing aids generally offer better sound quality and can be precisely programmed to meet the consumer's communication needs.

REFERENCES

American Speech-Language and Hearing Association (1989). Mental retardation and developmental disabilities curriculum guide for speech-language pathologists and audiologists. *ASHA, 31,* 94–96.

Benham-Dunster, R. A., & Dunster, J. R. (1985). Hearing loss in the developmentally handicapped: A comparison of three audiometric procedures. *The Journal of Auditory Research, 25,* 175–190.

Bess, F. H. & Humes, L. E. (1990). *Audiology: the fundamentals.* Baltimore: Williams & Wilkins.

Byers, V. W. & Bristow, D. C. (1990). Audiological evaluation of nonspeaking, physically challenged populations. *Ear and Hearing, 11*(5), 382–386.

Cornacchia, L., Vigliani., & Arpini, A. (1982). Comparison between brainstem-evoked response audiometry and behavioral audiometry in 270 infants and children. *Audiology, 21,* 359–363.

Crandell, C. C., & Roeser, R. J. (1993). Incidence of excessive impacted cerumen in individuals with mental retardation: a longitudinal investigation. *American Journal of Mental Retardation, 97,* 568–574.

Dahle, A. J., & McCollister, F. P. (1986). Hearing and otologic disorders in children with Down syndrome. *American Journal of Mental Deficiency, 90,* 636–642.

Decker, T. N., & Wilson, W. R. (1977). The use of visual reinforcement audiometry (VRA) with profound retarded residents. *Mental Retardation, 15,* 40–41.

Developmental Disabilities Assistance and Bill of Rights Act of 1990, Title 42, U.S.C. 6000–6083, *U. S. Statutes at Large, 104,* 1191–1204.

Diefendorf, A. O. (2002). Detection and assessment of hearing loss in infants and children. In J. Katz, (Ed.). *Handbook of clinical audiology* (5th ed.). New York: Lippincott Williams & Wilkins.

Don, M., & Kwong, B. (2002). Auditory brainstem response: Differential diagnosis. In J. Katz, (Ed.). *Handbook of clinical audiology* (5th ed.). New York: Lippincott Williams & Wilkins.

Evenhuis, H. M. (1995). Medical aspects of aging in a population with intellectual disability: II. Hearing impairment. *Journal of Intellectual Disability Research, 39,* 27–33.

Evenhuis, H. M. (1996). Dutch consensus on diagnosis and treatment of hearing impairment in children and adults with intellectual disability. *Journal of Intellectual Disability Research, 40,* 451–456.

Fisch, L. (1955). Deafness in cerebral palsied school children. *Lancet, 269,* 370–371.

Friedrich, B. W. (1985). The state of the art in audiologic evaluation and management. In E. Cherow, (Ed.). *Children and youth with developmental disabilities.* Washington, DC: Gallaudet College Press.

Fulton, R. T. & Lamb, L. E. (1972). Acoustic impedance and tympanometry with the retarded: A normative study. *Audiology, 11,* 199–208.

Gans, D. P., & Gans, K. D. (1993). Development of a hearing test protocol for profoundly involved multi-handicapped children. *Ear & Hearing, 14*(2), 128–140.

Gersh, E. S. (1991). Medical concerns and treatment. In E. Geralis, (Ed.), *Children with Cerebral Palsy*. Bethesda, MD: Woodbine House, Inc.

Green, K. W., & Margolis, R. H. (1983). Detection of hearing loss with ipsilateral acoustic reflex thresholds. *Audiology, 22*, 471–479.

Hall, J. W. (2000). *Handbook of otoacoustic emissions*. San Diego, CA: Singular Publishing.

Hannley, M. (1984). Immittance audiometry (pp. 57–83). In J. Jerger, (Ed.). *Hearing disorders in adults*. San Diego, CA: College-Hill.

Hur, J. J. (1997). Skills for independence for children with cerebral palsy: A comparative longitudinal study. *International Journal of Disability, Development and Education, 44*(3), 263–274.

Jerger, J., Burney, P., Mauldin, L., & Crump, B. (1974). Predicting hearing loss from the acoustic reflex. *Journal of Speech and Hearing Disorders, 39*, 11–22.

Keiser, H., Montague, J., Wold, D., Maune, S. & Pattison, D. (1981). Hearing loss of Down syndrome adults. *American Journal of Mental Deficiency, 85*(5), 467–472.

Kile, J. E. (1996). Audiologic assessment of children with Down syndrome. *American Journal of Audiology, 5*(1), 44–51.

Konstantareas, M. M., & Homatidis, S. (1987). Brief report: Ear infections in autistic and normal children. *Journal of Autism and Developmental Disorders, 17*, 585–594.

Kraus, N., Ozdamar, O., Stein, L., & Reed, N. (1984). Absent auditory brainstem response: Peripheral hearing loss or brainstem dysfunction. *Laryngoscope, 94*, 400–406.

Kuban, K.-C. K., & Leviton, A. (1994). Cerebral palsy. *The New England Journal of Medicine, 330*(3), 188–193.

Lancioni, G. E., & Coninx, F. (1995). A classical condition procedure for auditory testing: Air puff audiometry. *Scandinavian Audiology Supplement, 41*, 43–48.

Levine, M. (1971). Hearing problems and the cerebral palsy child. Paper presented to the Dental Guidance Council for Cerebral Palsy, New York.

Ling, D. (1978). Auditory coding and recording: An analysis of auditory training procedures for hearing impaired children. In M. Ross, & T. Giolas, (Eds.). *Auditory management of hearing impaired children*. Baltimore: University Park Press.

Lloyd, L. L., & Moore, E. J. (1972). Audiology (pp. 141–163). In J. Wortis, (Ed.). *Mental retardation: An annual review* (4th ed.). New York: Grune & Stratton.

Mandell, J. R. (2002). *Behavioral audiologic evaluation of infants and young children*. New York: Thieme Medical Publishers, Inc.

Maurizi, M., Altissimi, G. Ottaviani, F., Paludetti, G., & Bambini, M. (1982). Auditory brainstem responses (ABR) in the aged. *Scandinavian Audiology, 11*, 213–221.

Maurizi, M., Ottaviani, F., Paludetti, G., Almadori, G., Rosignoli, M., Tassoni, A. (1984). Middle-latency auditory components in response to clicks and low- and middle-latency tone pips (0.5–1 KHZ). *Audiology, 23*, 569–580.

Maurizi, M., Ottaviani, F., & Paludetti (1995). Objective methods of hearing assessment: An introduction. *Scandinavian Audiology Supplement 41*, 4–7.

Mazzoni, D. S., Ackley, R. S., & Nash, D. J. (1994). Abnormal pinna type and hearing loss correlations in Down syndrome. *Journal of Intellectual Disability Research, 38*, 549–560.

MCW Health Link. (2002). Health care for adults with Down syndrome. Retrieved from http://healthlink.mcw.edu/article/1001820316.html. Triangle Down syndrome network ear and hearing considerations for children with Down syndrome, accessed via www.triangledownsyndrome.org/ent.htm.

McCormick, B. (1995). History and state-of-the-art in behavioral methods for hearing assessment in low-functioning children. *Scandinavian Audiology Supplement, 41*, 31–35.

Molnar, G. E. (1985). *Paediatric rehabilitation*. Baltimore: Williams & Wilkins.

Mutch, L., Alberman, E., Hagberg, B., Kodama, K., & Perat, M. V. (1992). Cerebral palsy epidemiology: Where are we now and where are we going? *Devlopmental Medicine and Child Neurology, 34*, 547–551.

Mysak, E. D., (1971). Hearing disorders among the cerebral palsied. In L. E. Travis, (Ed.), *Handbook of Speech Pathology and Audiology* (pp. 678–679). New York: Appleton-Century-Crofts.

Nakano, T. (1966). Research hearing impairment in cerebral infantile palsied school children. *International Audiology, 5*, 159–161.

Niemeyer, W., & Sesterhenn, G. (1974). Calculating the hearing threshold from the stapedius reflex for different sound stimuli. *Audiology, 13*, 421–427.

Nelson, K. B. & Ellenberg, J. R. (1978). Epidemiology of cerebral palsy. *Advanced Neurology, 19*, 421–435.

Oyiborhoro, J. M. A. (1993, April). Impacted cerumen in a cerebral palsy population. Paper presented at the American Academy of Audiology Convention, Phoenix, Arizona.

Petrak, M. R. (2000, August). Integrating physiologic technologies for hearing evaluation in infants and small children: An overview. Unpublished handout: ICS Medical.

Pharaoh, P. O., Cooke, T., & Rosenbloom, L. (1989). Acquired cerebral palsy. *Archives of Disease in Childhood, 64*, 1013–1016.

Pruszewicz, A., Obrebowski, A. & Fgorzalewicz, B. (1977). Selected problems in the hearing, voice, and speech disturbances in the extrapyramidal form of cerebral palsy. *Folia Phoniatrica, 29*, 302–310.

Ray, C. (2002). Mental retardation and/or developmental disabilities. In J. Katz, (Ed.). *Handbook of clinical audiology* (5th ed.). New York: Lippincott Williams & Wilkins.

Rittmanic, P. A. (1971). The mentally retarded and mentally ill (pp. 369–404). In D. E. Rose, (Ed.). *Audiological assessment* (1st ed.). Englewood Cliffs, NJ: Prentice-Hall.

Ross, M., & Lerman, J. (1970). A picture identification test for hearing impaired children. *Journal of Speech and Hearing Research, 13*, 44–53.

Sanders, J. W., & Josey, A. F. (1970). Narrow-band noise audiometry for hard-to-test patients. *Journal of Speech and Hearing Research, 13*, 74–81.

Siegenthaler, B. M. (1987). Auditory problems (pp. 85–103). In E. T. McDonald, (Ed.): *Treating cerebral palsy: For clinicians by clinicians*. Austin, TX: Pro-Ed.

Smith, L. E., & Simmons, F. B. (1982). Accuracy of auditory brainstem evoked response with hearing level unknown. *Annals of Otology, Rhinolology, and Laryngology, 91*, 266–267.

Smyth, V. (1984). Successful auditory brainstem evoked response testing and test-age relationships in difficult-to-test children. *Australian Paediatric Journal, 20*, 115–117.

Sutton, G. J., Gleadle, P., & Rowe, S. J. (1996). Tympanometry and otoacoustic emissions in a cohort of special care neonates. *British Journal of Audiology, 30*(1), 9–17.

Swif, E. & Rosin, M. (1988). Communication profile in Down syndrome individuals. Presented at the annual convention of the Wisconsin Speech-Hearing-Language Association.

Talbott, C. B. (1987). A longitudinal study comparing responses of hearing-impaired infants to pure tones using visual reinforcement and play audiometry. *Ear & Hearing, 8,* 175–179.

Thompson, G., & Weber, B. A. (1974). Responses of infants and young children to behavioral observation audiometry (BOA). *Journal of Speech and Hearing Disorders, 39,* 140–147.

Thompson, G., Wilson, W. R. & Moore, J. M. (1979). Application of visual reinforcement audiometry (VRA) to low-functioning children. *Journal of Speech Hearing Disorder, 44,* 80–90.

Van Schrojenstein Lantman-DeValk, H. M. J., Haveman, M. J., Maaskant, M. A., Kessela, A. G. H., Urlings, H. F. J., & Sturmans, F. (1994). The need for assessment of sensory functioning in aging people with mental handicaps. *Journal of Intellectual Disability Research, 38,* 289–298.

Widen, J. E., & O'Grady, G. M. (2002). Using visual reinforcement audiometry in the assessment of hearing infants. *The Hearing Journal,* 55, 11.

Wilber, L. A. (2002). Transducers for audiologic testing (pp. 88–95). In J. Katz, (Ed.). *Handbook of clinical audiology* (5th ed.). Baltimore: Williams & Wilkins.

Worthington, D. W., & Peters, J. F. (1980). Quantifiable hearing and no ABR: Paradox or error? *Ear & Hearing, 1,* 281–285.

Young, C. V. (1994). Developmental disabilities (pp. 521–533). In J. Katz, (Ed.). *Handbook of clinical audiology* (4th ed.). Baltimore: Williams & Wilkins.

SELECTED READINGS

Bleck, E. E. (1979). *Orthopaedic management of cerebral palsy.* Philadelphia: W.B. Saunders.

Flexer, C., & Gans, D. P. (1985). Comparative evaluation of the auditory responsiveness of normal infants and profoundly multi handicapped children. *Journal of Speech and Hearing Research, 28,* 163–168.

Gans, D. P., & Flexer, C. (1982). Observer bias in the hearing testing of profoundly involved multiply handicapped children. *Ear & Hearing, 3,* 309–313.

Graham, L., Martin, F., & Bernstein, M. (1989). A survey of the procedures used in Texas for the audiological evaluation of severely to profoundly multi-handicapped children. *Texas Journal of Speech Pathology and Audiology, 15,* 47–48.

Jerger, J., & Hayes, D. (1976). The cross-check principle in pediatric audiometry. *Archives of Otology, 102,* 614–620.

Liden, G., & Kankkunen, A. (1969). Visual reinforcement audiometry. *Acta Otolaryngology, 67,* 281–292.

Sonksen, P. M. (1979). Sound and the visually handicapped baby. *Child Health and Development, 5,* 413–420.

Schopler, E., Reichler, R. J., DeVellis, R. F., & Daly, K. (1980). Objective classification of childhood autism: Childhood autism rating scale. *Journal of Autism and Developmental Disorders, 10,* 91–103.

Suzuki, T., & Ogiba, Y. (1961). Conditioned orientation reflex audiometry. *Journal of Speech and Hearing Disorders, 39,* 140–147.

Syndulko, K., Cohen, S. N., Pettler-Jennings, P., Shah, J., Friedman, A., Potvin, A. R., & Tourtellotte, W. W. (1984). P300 and neurocognitive function in neurologic patients (pp. 441–445). In R. H. Noder & C. Barber (Eds.). *Evoked potentials II: The Second International Evoked Potentials Symposium.* Boston: Butterworth.

Tweedie, D. (1975). Videoaudiometry: A possible procedure for "difficult-to-test" populations: *Volta Review, 77,* 109–134.

CHAPTER 3

HIV/AIDS

John M.A. Oyiborhoro, Ed.D., F.A.A.A., CCC-A
Boro Audiology Clinic
Brooklyn, NY
and
National Institute for People with Disabilities
New York, NY

Modes of Transmission of HIV
HIV Infection and AIDS-Related Pathologic
   Conditions
      Some Causes of AIDS-Related Diseases/Lesions
      Auditory Disorders Associated with AIDS
      Conductive Auditory Pathologic Conditions
      Causes of Sensorineural Hearing Loss in
         HIV-Positive Individuals and
         Patients with AIDS
      Retrocochlear Pathologic Conditions
      Auditory P300 Response
Management
References
Suggested Readings

Human immunodeficiency virus (HIV) infection and acquired immune deficiency syndrome (AIDS) existed for decades before 1981 when the occurrence of AIDS became an epidemic (Larsen, 1998). AIDS is undoubtedly one of world's most dreaded killer diseases. Since 1981 when the U.S. Centers for Disease Control and Prevention (CDC) in Atlanta reported and described cases of HIV infection and patients living with AIDS (CDC, 1981a), HIV infection and the disease AIDS have spread rather rapidly throughout the world with devastating consequences along the way. AIDS is especially widespread in developing countries that are the least able to economically and technologically combat and arrest a spread of the epidemic. AIDS has decimated populations and destroyed family units in these developing countries, especially in sub-Saharan Africa where the impact has been most severe. About 90% of new HIV infections each year occur in developing countries (Pivot, 1997).

The initial cases of AIDS-related diseases were reported in homosexual men who presented an unusual form of pneumonia caused by *Pneumocystis carinii,* Kaposi's sarcoma, and other infections caused by opportunistic pathogens (CDC, 1981b). The CDC (1981c) then defined AIDS as a disease that is at least moderately predictive of a defect in cell-mediated immunity occurring in a person with no known cause for diminished resistance to the disease. According to the CDC, such diseases include Kaposi's sarcoma, *Pneumocystis carinii* pneumonia, and serious opportunistic infections.

HIV-infected individuals and patients living with AIDS experience a wide spectrum of AIDS-related diseases and disabilities, some directly as a result of HIV infection and others indirectly from the treatment of AIDS itself or the prophylactic action of HIV treatment drugs.

Some of the disabling conditions experienced by HIV-1–infected individuals and patients with AIDS include cognitive and motor function deficits (Flower & Sooy, 1987; Sahakia et al., 1995). Of more interest to us are the auditory manifestations of AIDS that have been well documented in the literature (Kohan, Rothstein, & Cohen, 1988; Lalwani & Sooy, 1992; Moazzez & Alvi, 1998; Morris & Prasad, 1990; Rarey, 1990; Soucek & Michaels, 1996). The auditory manifestations include, but are not limited to, the following conditions and audiologic evaluation outcomes: otitis externa, serous and chronic otitis media, eustachian tube dysfunction, sensorineural hearing loss, vertigo, gait problems, conductive hearing loss, sudden or progressive sensorineural hearing loss, tinnitus, Kaposi's sarcoma, nasopharyngeal mass, central nervous system (CNS) complications, auditory brainstem response (ABR) abnormalities, and otoacoustic emissions (OAE) abnormalities. We will return to manifestations of AIDS later in this chapter, but first we will examine the nature of the killer HIV, the way it is transmitted, and then its pathogenic/histopathogenic consequences.

Viruses, in general, are nonliving organisms that are composed of protein molecules called ribonucleic acid (RNA) or deoxyribonucleic acid (DNA). A virus is made up of either RNA or DNA, not a combination of both. A virus made of RNA protein molecules is referred to as a retrovirus. This virus contains a self-regulatory gene that enables it to self-replicate (producing several copies of itself) and also causes its pathogenetic actions as it attacks and attaches itself to the host cell.

The human immune system contains protective fighting cells (phagocytes). These cells search and destroy invading killer cells (pathogens) to enable the human body to maintain good health. However, if the immune system is compromised, then other opportunistic pathogens that hitherto were not harmful become pathogenic and, thus, harmful. HIV has a special affinity for human T-helper lymphocytes. The T-helper lymphocyte cells induce the most immunogenic actions to fight off invading foreign killer cells. The pathogenic action of HIV tends to deplete T-helper lymphocyte cell counts. Reduced T-helper lymphocyte cell counts render the immune system weak, less capable of defending itself, and prone to opportunistic attack by other pathogens.

MODES OF TRANSMISSION OF HIV

Sources of transmission of HIV are displayed in Table 3.1. The primary mode of transmission is through unprotected sexual contact, especially by receptive anal intercourse. HIV is also transmitted through transfusion of infected blood; needle-sharing among intravenous drug abusers; and transplacental, perinatal (i.e., during natural delivery), or postnatal (during breast feeding) transmittal from an HIV-infected mother to her child. It has been suggested that about 50% of people infected with HIV will develop full-blown AIDS within 10 years (Watson, 1996). However, with the new drugs now available, people are living much longer and more productive lives than ever before because the development of full-blown AIDS is being delayed considerably.

Table 3.1

People at Risk of Contracting HIV Infection and AIDS

1. Sexually active homosexual men
2. Bisexual men and their partners (male/female)
3. Intravenous drug users (who share needles)
4. Heterosexual men and women (with multiple partners)
5. People who receive blood transfusions (with unscreened blood)
6. People who take blood products (made from tainted blood)
7. People who have sexual contacts with HIV-infected individuals or patients with AIDS
8. Newborns of HIV-infected mothers
9. Immigrants from areas with many cases of AIDS.

Adapted from Cooper, P. G. (2000). AIDS: Risk factors and prevention of transmission. Pamphlet: Gale Group.

HIV INFECTION AND AIDS-RELATED PATHOLOGIC CONDITIONS

Watson (1996) listed three main areas into which indicators of AIDS as a disease can be classified. They are (1) infectious diseases, (2) neoplastic diseases, and (3) others.

First, AIDS-related infectious diseases include, but are by no means limited to, *P. carinii* pneumonia (more than 60% of patients with AIDS develop this disease), cytomegalovirus retinitis, esophageal candidiasis, cryptosporidiosis, and isosporiasis; all of these conditions are accompanied by diarrhea persisting for more than 1 month and toxoplasmosis of the brain. Second, neoplastic disease forms include Kaposi's sarcoma, which is described as the most common malignant tumor and manifestation in patients with AIDS, primary lymphoma of the brain, and non-Hodgkin's lymphoma. Third, other indicators of AIDS include HIV encephalopathy or what is also referred to as AIDS dementia, the HIV wasting syndrome, and a CD4 count of less than 200 T-helper lymphocytes/mm^3 (a CD4 count of 1000 cells/mm^3 represents an absolute helper lymphocyte count). When the CD4 count is less than 200/mm^3, the development of full-blown AIDS in the HIV-infected individual is imminent if prophylactic action is not taken immediately.

Some Causes of AIDS-Related Diseases/Lesions

Infections in HIV-infected individuals are caused by opportunistic pathogens, which may be viruses, fungi, or bacteria. In individuals with noncompromised immune systems, these numerous pathogens can be found in the body but are not harmful because they are unable to infect their host cells. If the immune system is compromised, infection may occur because of the opportunity provided by the weakened or altered physiologic condition of the host.

HIV pathogenic activities weaken or suppress the immune system in infected individuals. This provides the opportunity for otherwise nonharmful pathogens to become pathogenic by attacking host cells, thus causing infections and life-threatening complications (Grimaldi et al., 1993; Kohan et al., 1988; Pappas, Roland, Lin, Lai, & Hillman, 1995). Hearing impairment is one of the manifestations associated with HIV infection and AIDS, which is caused by the actions of opportunistic pathogens. These pathogens include cytomegalovirus (CMV), which is considered to be the most opportunistic pathogen, *P. carinii, Staphylococcus aureus, Mycobacterium tuberculosis,* and *Toxoplasma gondii.* Other infections, such as herpes simplex, Ramsay Hunt syndrome, or herpes zoster oticus, caused by opportunistic pathogens are also seen (Bankaitis & Keith, 1995; Grimaldi et al., 1993; Pappas et al., 1995). Individuals with Ramsay Hunt syndrome or herpes zoster oticus may have ipsilateral facial paralysis, sensorineural hearing loss, tinnitus, and vertigo (Watson, 1996). Although most forms of otitis media that occur in HIV-infected and non–HIV-infected individuals and patients with AIDS are caused by the usual pathogens such as *Streptococcus pneumoniae, Haemophilus influenzae,* and *Moraxella catarrhalis* (Gherman, Ward, & Bassis, 1998; Kohan, Hammerschlag, & Holliday, 1990; Lalwani & Sooy, 1992), otitis media and mastoiditis caused by *P. carinii* have been reported as opportunistic infections that are unique to patients with AIDS (Breda, Hammershlag, Gigliotti, & Schinella, 1998; Gherman et al., 1988; Morris & Prasad, 1990; Watson, 1996). Otitis media may also result from eustachian tube dysfunction caused by obstructions from AIDS-related nasopharyngeal tumors (Lalwani & Sooy, 1992; Moazzez & Alvi, 1998).

Auditory Disorders Associated with AIDS

With better antiretroviral drugs and management of people with HIV infection and AIDS, they are living longer, but mortality from AIDS remains at nearly 100% (Moazzez & Alvi, 1998). In addition to living longer, HIV-infected individuals can have productive lives. The spectrum of disorders associated with HIV-1 infection and AIDS calls for a multidisciplinary approach and therefore the involvement of practitioners for other specialties and subspecialties such as audiology, speech-language pathology, otolaryngology, neurology, ophthalmology, psychiatry, and gastroenterology (Larsen, 1998). To function well as a team player, the audiologist should be knowledgeable and be aware of the auditory anomalies that are associated with HIV infection and AIDS and the management roles that might be needed.

Auditory disorders and their audiologic correlates associated with HIV/AIDS are displayed in Table 3.2. As can be observed, auditory disorders and complaints constitute a significant aspect of the consequences of HIV infection and AIDS. Auditory disorders associated with HIV/ AIDS may not always be caused directly by HIV, but occur as a result of the pathogenic actions of the virus.

The occurrence of conductive, sensorineural, and retrocochlear pathologic conditions in HIV infected individuals and patients living with AIDS is well documented (Breda et al., 1988; Gherman et al., 1988; Grimaldi et al., 1993; Kohan et al., 1988; Real, Thomas, & Gerwin, 1987; Smith & Canalis, 1989; Soucek & Michaels, 1996; Timon & Walsh, 1989). However, because of more life-threatening events due to complications caused by opportunistic infections in HIV-infected individuals and patients with AIDS, the auditory pathologic conditions and their audiologic correlates often take a secondary position and may therefore be under-reported so their occurrence may be higher than studies show (Bankaitis & Keith, 1995; Kwartler et al., 1991; Soucek & Michaels, 1996; Timon & Walsh, 1989).

CONDUCTIVE AUDITORY PATHOLOGIC CONDITIONS

Auditory disorders of the outer and middle ear due to complications of HIV infection include otitis externa; aural polyps; Kaposi's sarcoma; non-Hodgkin's lymphoma; eustachian tube dysfunction; serous, chronic, and acute otitis media; tympanic membrane perforation; ossicular discontinuity; cholesteatoma; and nasopharyngeal neoplasms (Breda et al., 1988; Kohan et al., 1988; Lalwani & Sooy, 1992; Moazzez & Alvi, 1998; Rarey, 1990). These disease processes affect audiologic findings. It is important therefore for the audiologist to be knowledgeable about the patient's pathophysiology and possible audiologic outcomes as a result of their manifestation in the auditory mechanism.

Otitis externa is a malignant disease process that affects the cartilaginous portion of the external auditory canal in HIV-infected individuals. Chronic otitis externa infection is usually caused by *Pseudomonas aeruginosa* (Moazzez & Alvi, 1998). The incidence of otitis externa in individuals with AIDS is generally not higher than in

Table 3.2

Auditory Disorders Associated with HIV/AIDS

External Ear	Middle Ear	Inner Ear	CNS
Otitis externa	Eustachian tube dysfunction	Vertigo	Retrocochlear pathologic conditions
Aural polyps	Serous/acute otitis media	Imbalance	VII cranial nerve (facial) palsy
Kaposi's sarcoma	Cholesteatoma	Tinnitus	VIII cranial nerve (vestibulocochlear bundle) neuropathy
Non-Hodgkin's lymphoma	Nasopharyngeal tumors	Endolymphatic hydrops	Dementia
Conductive hearing loss	Ossicular discontinuity	Abnormal ABR	Abnormal P300 response
	Abnormal OAE	Abnormal OAE	
	Tympanic membrane perforation	Sudden and/or progressive Sensorineural hearing loss	
	Conductive hearing loss	Sensorineural hearing loss (SNHL)	

individuals with noncompromised immune systems (Kohan et al., 1988; Lalwani & Sooy, 1992). Thus it has been suggested that otitis externa is perhaps not exactly a manifestation of AIDS, but rather that it may represent an incidental auditory disorder that is present in HIV-positive individuals and persons with AIDS (Morris & Prasad, 1990). However, Moazzez and Alvi (1988) suggested that immunocompromised individuals with HIV/AIDS may be more predisposed to malignant otitis externa. In addition to reporting severe progressive pain, individuals with otitis externa infection also complain of a hearing loss (Moazzez & Alvi, 1998). This may possibly be conductive because of the presence of excessive or impacted and microbe-infested purulent debris in the external ear canal. Medical referral should be made for ear canal débridement and antibiotic treatment (Moazzez & Alvi, 1998; Morris & Prasad, 1990).

Kaposi's sarcoma is considered to be the most common malignant tumor in immunocompromised individuals with AIDS, about 20,000 times more common than in the nonimmunocompromised population (Moazzez & Alvi, 1998; Noel et al., 1996). Kaposi's sarcoma occurs mostly in the external ear of individuals with AIDS. Because of the involvement of the pinna, ear canal, tympanic membrane, eustachian tube, and the nasopharynx, Kaposi's sarcoma causes conductive hearing loss (Lalwani & Sooy, 1988; Moazzez & Alvi, 1998; Morris & Prasad, 1990).

Many adults with AIDS often present serous otitis media with effusion (i.e., without signs of inflammation of the middle ear), an occurrence more common than that in the general population (Lalwani & Sooy, 1988). Serous otitis media with effusion or secretory otitis media can be caused by eustachian tube dysfunction resulting from nasopharyngeal tumors (Morris & Prasad, 1990; Stern, Lin, & Lucente, 1990).

Chronic otitis media with or without cholesteatoma is more common in immunocompromised persons with AIDS than in the general population (Moazzez & Alvi, 1998). Common causes of chronic otitis media are opportunistic infections caused by *S. pneumoniae, H. influenza,* and *M. catarrhalis.* Chronic otitis media and mastoiditis caused by opportunistic pathogenic action of *P. carinii* are not common. However, according to Lalwani and Sooy (1992), *P. carinii,* which is found in aural polyps in the external ear canal, can spread to the middle ear space via the eustachian tube from an infected nasopharynx. Chronic ear pain and mixed hearing loss usually accompany chronic otitis media. Audiologic findings typically yield abnormal tympanograms and significantly abnormal OAEs.

Depending on the hearing loss criteria used, studies have shown that the incidence of sensorineural hearing loss in HIV-positive individuals and patients with AIDS is 20–69% (Grimaldi et al., 1993; Lalwani & Sooy, 1992; Sooy, 1987; Soucek & Michaels, 1996). Using a hearing loss criterion of worse than 25 dB hearing sensitivity, Lalwani & Sooy (1992) found a 45% incidence of sensorineural hearing impairment in their study, which involved immunocompromised patients with AIDS. In a separate study Soucek and Michaels (1996) reported an even higher incidence of sensorineural hearing impairment of 69% in their subjects with AIDS, but they used the criterion of a worse than 20 dB hearing loss. According to Sooy (1987), sensorineural hearing loss appears to be more prevalent than conductive hearing loss in HIV-infected persons. This finding should be of concern to both HIV-positive individuals and patients with AIDS and their caregivers, because, except in few instances of fluctuating sensorineural hearing loss such as in Ménière's disease, sensorineural hearing impairment is permanent. Medical intervention is essentially preventive, because there is no known medical treatment for hearing deficiencies caused by cochlear lesions or damage to the hair cells, which results in sensorineural hearing loss.

CAUSES OF SENSORINEURAL HEARING LOSS IN HIV-POSITIVE INDIVIDUALS AND PATIENTS WITH AIDS

There are three sources of AIDS-related sensorineural hearing impairment as suggested by Soucek and Michaels (1998): (1) AIDS-related cochlear lesions, (2) ototoxicity caused by prescribed prophylactic drugs or medications used in the treatment of AIDS-related disease conditions, and (3) AIDS-related lesions of the auditory pathway involving the CNS.

AIDS-Related Cochlear Lesions

A weakened immune system renders the patient with AIDS more prone to opportunistic infections that cause meningitis. Meningitis is considered to be one of the causes of cochlear lesions, which result in sensorineural hearing loss in patients with AIDS (Kohan et al., 1988; Morris & Prasad, 1990). Some types of meningitis caused by opportunistic pathogens are cryptococcal meningitis, tuberculous meningitis, bacterial and viral meningitis, and neurosyphilis (Kohan et al., 1988; Kwartler et al., 1991). Sudden sensorineural hearing loss has been associated with cryptococcal meningitis (Kwartler et al., 1991).

In addition to meningogenic causes for sensorineural hearing loss, CMV infection constitutes another major cause of cochlear lesions in patients with AIDS. CMV infection of the temporal bone in patients with AIDS impairs cochlear function by involving the efferent innervation to the cochlea (Soucek & Michaels, 1996) with inflammation of the internal auditory canal through which the efferent fibers of the vestibulocochlear nerve bundle run.

Ototoxicity from AIDS-Related Drug Therapy

Ototoxicity from drugs used either as prophylactic treatment of HIV infection and/or neoplasms in patients with AIDS is another possible cause of cochlear lesions and sensorineural hearing loss (Marra et al., 1997). *Ototoxicity* is defined as chemically induced injury to the inner ear that causes varying degrees of sensorineural hearing loss (Bankaitis & Keith, 1995).

Medical treatment of HIV infection and AIDS relies heavily on use of drug therapy. The ototoxic effects of new antiretrovial drugs that are used on an experimental basis for the treatment of patients with AIDS are not known. Some of these drugs include, but are not limited to, azidothymidine, acyclovir, ethambutol, isoniazid, ganciclovir, trimethoprim-sulfamethoxazole, isoprenaline, flucytosine, and zidovudine (Kohan et al., 1990; Marra et al., 1997; Soucek & Michaels, 1996). Because of the life-threatening nature of complications of AIDS, known ototoxic, antifungal drugs such as amphotericin B, aminoglycoside antibiotics, and antineoplastic drugs such as erythromycin are often used to treat AIDS-related complications or are used as preventive measures in HIV-positive persons (Bankaitis & Keith, 1995).

Results from a study by Kohan et al. (1988) showed that sensorineural hearing loss present in their subjects with AIDS could only be explained by their exposure to known ototoxic antibiotics such as streptomycin and aminoglycosides. Histopathologic findings suggest that sensorineural hearing impairment in patients with AIDS may be due in part to ototoxic damage to the cochlea, which is manifested in the loss of cochlear outer hair cells (Soucek & Michaels, 1996).

AIDS–Related Lesions of the Auditory Pathway of the CNS

In immunocompromised patients with AIDS, the CNS is prone to opportunistic infections as well as to development of neoplasms in the central auditory pathway (Petito et al., 1986). Soucek and Michaels (1996) suggested that damage to the central auditory pathways could possibly cause sensorineural hearing impairment. Neurophysiologic studies of patients with AIDS who have sudden bilateral sensorineural hearing loss revealed bilateral involvement of both branches of the vestibulocochlear cranial nerves (Grimaldi et al., 1993; Kwartler et al., 1991; Real et al., 1987). Real et al. (1987) investigated the possible cause of sudden sensorineural hearing impairment in a male homosexual with AIDS, who was exposed to opportunistic infections and later developed an intracerebral hemorrhage. They concluded that the sensorineural hearing loss in their patients with AIDS was perhaps due to involvement of the acoustic cranial nerve or to cryptococcal meningitis. Thus acoustic cranial nerve neuropathy associated with HIV infection can cause sensorineural hearing loss.

Many patients with AIDS often present vertigo and other vestibular abnormalities such as imbalance, ataxia, and nausea. As indicated earlier under causes of sensorineural hearing loss, vestibular abnormalities in patients with AIDS are possibly due to involvement of the vestibulocochlear cranial nerve bundle (Grimaldi et al., 1993; Kwartler et al., 1991) resulting from neoplasmic growths or opportunistic infection that affects the internal auditory meatus.

RETROCOCHLEAR PATHOLOGIC CONDITIONS

One direct effect of HIV infection on the CNS is the development of retrocochlear pathologic conditions that have an impact on audiologic outcomes, especially ABR findings (Lalwani & Sooy, 1992). Significantly abnormal ABR findings obtained with HIV-positive individuals and patients with AIDS have been attributed to complications of HIV infection and AIDS (Birchall, Wight, French, Cockbain, & Smith, 1992; Welkoborsky & Lowitzsch, 1992). ABR measures the sequence of neural activity from the vestibulocochlear nerve bundle to the pons level of the brainstem. Waves I and II are generated from the acoustic nerve whereas other waves are generated from other actions of the brainstem. ABR is quite sensitive and reliable in assessing and detecting pathologic conditions of the acoustic nerve and the brainstem such as acoustic neuromas, demyelinating and degenerative diseases, and vascular lesions (Bankaitis & Keith, 1995). ABR findings are usually interpreted on the basis of an analysis of absolute latencies of waves I, II, and V; the interpeak latencies of waves I–III, III–V, and I–V; and the amplitude ratio of waves V:I, which are then compared with normative test data (Clemins & McGee, 1979; Clemins & Mitchell, 1977; Daly, Roeser, Aung, & Daly, 1997). These normative data sometimes vary from one clinic to another due to their specific clinical procedures.

HIV/AIDS-related pathologic conditions in the central auditory pathway of CNS such as acoustic neuroma and cryptococcal meningitis, which often involves the vestibulocochlear nerve bundle, yield abnormal ABRs that are observed as delays in interpeak latencies and amplitudes of individual waves. Results from several studies (Birchall et al., 1992; Lalwani & Sooy, 1992; Welkoborsky & Lowitzsch, 1992) indicate that HIV infection and complications of AIDS directly compromise the integrity of ABR readings with significant delays at interpeak latencies between waves III and V. It should be noted, however, that the conclusions of some studies are contradictory. Not all HIV-infected patients who have not developed full-blown AIDS present abnormal ABR findings (Iragui, Kalmijin, Thal, Grant, & HNRC Group, 1994; Madriz & Herrera, 1995; Ragazzoni et al., 1993). According to Bankaitis and Keith (1995), the normal ABR readings recorded in some HIV-infected patients may be due in part to nonuniform procedures and techniques, which are used in various clinics and studies. For instance, in demyelinating disease processes, a change in ABR click rates from slower to faster has been shown to yield abnormal ABR findings even when ABR responses might have appeared normal at lower click rates (Antonelli et al., 1998). Neurophysiologic and neuropathologic studies (Anders, Guerra, Tomiyasu, Verity, & Vinters, 1986; Grimaldi et al., 1993; Rostad, Sumi, Shaw, Olson, & McDougall, 1987; Simpson & Bender, 1988) reveal that

HIV infection induces neuropathologic alterations, especially subcortical demyelination (as in leukoencephalopathy) of portions of the medulla pons and mid brain. Leukoencephalopathy is a common manifestation in patients with full-blown AIDS. Demyelination in these areas (medulla, pons, and mid-brain) interferes with the temporal synchronization of neural activity and transmission of neural information through the central auditory pathways in HIV-infected individuals and patients with AIDS (Rostad et al., 1987), resulting in significantly abnormal ABR findings.

AUDITORY P300 RESPONSE

AIDS-related dementia is seen in up to 87% of patients with AIDS (Price et al., 1988) as a result of the involvement of subcortical and cortical levels of the CNS from opportunistic infections. The P300 response develops approximately 300 ms after presentation of auditory stimulus and is generated at the medial temporal lobe level, unlike ABR, which develops approximately 10 ms after a presentation auditory stimulus. A P300 response is thought to be generated at the medial temporal lobe level and corresponds to various cognitive processing, which requires short-term memory and the mental speed essential in decision making (Ford, Mohs, Pfefferbaum, & Kopell., 1980). Studies involving immunocompromised HIV-positive individuals and patients with AIDS reveal abnormal increases in P300 response latencies, suggesting cortical involvement in this population (St. Claire, Blackwood, & Christie, 1985). These findings should not be considered conclusive because there have been patients in whom the presence of dementias such as those of the Alzheimer type has yielded normal P300 responses (Syndulko et al., 1984). Audiologic evaluation of HIV-infected individuals and patients with AIDS should include a test battery approach composed of comprehensive assessment components that include, but are not limited to, pure tone and speech audiometry, immittance measurements, acoustic reflexes, OAE, and ABR audiometry. The focus of these test procedures should be on exploring alterations of the external middle and inner ear as well as subcortical and cortical portions of the central auditory pathway due to the pathogenic actions of HIV and AIDS-related complications.

The prevalence of both conductive and sensorineural hearing impairments in HIV-infected individuals and patients with AIDS is documented (Gherman et al., 1988; Kohan et al., 1988; Real et al., 1987). The incidence of conductive hearing loss is reported to be less than that of sensorineural hearing impairment in this population (Sooy, 1987). The causes of sensorineural hearing impairment are multifaceted and have been associated with ototoxicity of the drugs used for prophylactic treatment of HIV-infected persons and AIDS-related lesions of the cochlea and central auditory pathway of the CNS, such as acoustic cranial nerve neuropathy (Soucek & Michaels, 1998).

Conductive hearing impairment in HIV-positive individuals and patients with AIDS is documented to be caused by otitis externa; Kaposi's sarcoma; polyps in the external auditory meatus; serous, chronic, or acute otitis media; and eustachian tube dysfunction due to nasopharyngeal neoplasms (Gherman et al., 1988; Kohan et al., 1988). The causes of retrocochlear pathologic conditions in patients with AIDS are similar to those of sensorineural hearing loss because AIDS-related opportunistic infections and neoplastic growths in the central auditory pathway, which cause cochlear alterations, also produce peripheral vestibular anomalies as well as lesions in the CNS. These lesions often produce abnormal ABR and P300 responses.

MANAGEMENT

Aural rehabilitation involves hearing aid evaluation and fitting if the degree of hearing loss or hearing handicap makes hearing aid use appropriate. For patients with AIDS who present retrocochlear disorders such as AIDS-related dementia, Bankaitis and Keith (1995) suggested administering central auditory processing tests to assess functional auditory processing skills and better plan and institute appropriate management and rehabilitation strategies. For instance, HIV-infected individuals and patients with AIDS who recently experienced a significant sudden sensorineural hearing loss, have an impaired CNS, and/or have poor central auditory processing skills that affect speech and language may benefit from amplification as well as augmentative and alternative communication.

REFERENCES

Anders, K., Guerra, W. F., Tomiyasu, U., Verity, M. A., & Vinters, H. A. (1986). The neuropathology of AIDS. UCLA experience and review. *American Journal of Pathology, 124,* 537–558.

Antonelli, A. R., Bonfioli, R. F., Cappiello, J., Peretti, G., Zanetti, D., & Capra, R. (1988). Auditory evoked potential, test battery related to magnetic resonance imaging for multiple sclerosis patients. *Scandinavian Audiology Supplement, 30,* 191–196.

Bankaitis, A. E., & Keith, R. W. (1995). Audiological changes associated with HIV infection. *Ear Nose and Throat Journal, 75,* 353–359.

Birchall, M., Wight, R., French, P., Cockbain, Z., & Smith, S. J. (1992). Auditory function in patients infected with human immunodeficiency virus. *Clinical Otolaryngology, 17,* 117–121.

Breda, S. D., Hammershlag, P. E., Gigliotti, F., & Schinella, R. (1988). *Pneumocystis carinii* in the temporal bone as a primary manifestation of the acquired immunodeficiency syndrome. *Annals of Otology, Rhinology, and Laryngology, 97,* 427–431.

Centers for Disease Control. (1981a). *Pneumocystis* pneumonia—Los Angeles. *Morbidity and Mortality Weekly Report, 30*(21), 250–252.

Centers for Disease Control. (1981b). Kaposi's sarcoma and pneumonia among homosexual men—New York City and California. *Morbidity and Morality Weekly Report, 30*(33), 305–308.

Centers for Disease Control. (1981c). Update on acquired immune deficiency syndrome (AIDS) United States. *Morbidity and Mortality Weekly Report, 31*(37), 507–514.

Clemins, J. D., & McGee, T. (1979). Brainstem electric response audiometry in the differential diagnosis of acoustic tumors. *Laryngoscope, 89,* 31–42.

Clemins, J. D., & Mitchell, C. (1997). Electrocochleography and brainstem responses used in the diagnosis of acoustic tumors. *Journal of Otolaryngology, 6,* 447–458.

Cooper, P. G. (2002). AIDS: Risk factors and prevention of transmission. Pamphlet: Gale Group (A Thomson Corporation Company).

Daly, D. M., Roeser, R. J., Aung, M. H., & Daly, D. D. (1997). Early evoked potentials in patients with acoustic neuroma. *Electroencephalography and Clinical Neurophysiology, 43,* 151–159.

Flower, W. M., & Sooy, C. D. (1987). AIDS: An introduction for speech-language pathologists and audiologists *ASHA, 29*(11), 25–30.

Ford, J. M., Mohs, R. C., Pfefferbaum, A., & Kopell, B. S. (1980). On the utility of P3 latency and RT for studying cognitive processes. *Progress in Brain Research, 54,* 661–668.

Gherman, C. R., Ward, R. R., & Bassis, M. L. (1988). *Pneumocystis carinii* otitis media and mastoiditis as the initial manifestation of the acquired immunodeficiency syndrome. *American Journal of Medicine, 85,* 250–252.

Grimaldi, L. M., Luzi, L., Martino, G. V., Furlan, R., Nemni, R., Antonelli, A., et al. (1993). Bilateral eighth cranial nerve neuropathy in human immunodeficiency virus infection. *Journal of Neurology, 240,* 363–366.

Iragui, V. J., Kalmijin, J., Thal, L. J., Grant, I., & HNRC Group. (1994). Neurological dysfunction in asymptomatic HIV-I infected men: Evidence from evoked potentials. *Electroencephalography and Clinical Neurophysiology, 92,* 1–10.

Kohan, D., Hammerschlag, P. E., & Holliday, R. A. (1990). Otologic disease in AIDS patients: CT correlation. *Laryngoscope, 100,* 1326–1330.

Kohan, D., Rothstein, S. G., & Cohen, N. L. (1988). Otologic disease in patients with acquired immunodeficiency syndrome. *Annals of Otology Rhinology, and Laryngology, 97,* 636–640.

Kwartler, J. A., Linthicum, F. H., Jahn, A. F., & Hawke, M. (1991). Sudden hearing loss due to AIDS related cryptococcal meningitis. A temporal bone study. *Otolaryngology—Head & Neck Surgery, 104,* 265–269.

Lalwani, A. K., & Sooy, C. D. (1992). Otologic manifestations of acquired immunodeficiency syndrome. *The Otolaryngological Clinics of North America, 25,* 1183–1198.

Larsen, C. R. (1998). *HIV-1 and communication disorders: What speech and hearing professionals need to know.* San Diego, CA: Singular.

Madriz, J. J., & Herrera, G. (1995). Human immunodeficiency virus and acquired immune deficiency syndrome AIDS-related hearing disorders. *Journal of the American Academy of Audiology, 6,* 358–364.

Marra, C. M., Weckin, H. A., Longstreth, W. T., Jr., Rees, T. S., Syapin, C. L., & Gates, G. A. (1997). Hearing loss and antiretroviral therapy in patients infected with HIV-1. *Archives of Neurology, 54,* 407–410.

Moazzez, A. H., & Alvi, A. (1998). Head and neck manifestations of AIDS in adults. *American Family Physician, 57,* 1813–1822.

Morris, M. S., & Prasad, S. (1990). Otologic disease in the acquired immunodeficiency syndrome. *Ear, Nose, & Throat Journal, 69,* 451–453.

Noel, J. C., Hermans, P., Andre, J., Fayt, I., Simonart, T., Verhest, A., et al. (1996). Herpes virus-like DNA sequences and Kaposi's sarcoma: Relationship with epidemiology, clinical spectrum, and histologic features. *Cancer, 77,* 2132–2136.

Pappas, Jr., D. G., Roland, Jr., J. T., Lim, J., Lai, A., & Hillman, D. E. (1995). Ultrastructural findings in the vestibular end-organs of AIDS cases. *American Journal of Otology, 16,* 140–145.

Petito, C. K., Cho, E. S., Lemann, W., Navia, B. A., & Price, R. W. (1986). Neuropathology of acquired immunodeficiency syndrome (AIDS): An autopsy review. *Journal of Neuropathology and Experimental Neurology, 45,* 635–646.

Pivot, P. (1997, September–October). Global epidemiology of HIV infection. Paper presented at the 37th Interscience Conference on Antimicrobial Agents and Chemotherapy (ICAAC), Toronto, Ontario, Canada.

Price, R. W., Brew, B., Sidtis, J., Rosenblum, M., Scheck, A. C., & Cleary, P. (1988). The brain in AIDS: Central nervous system HIV-1 infection and AIDS dementia complex. *Science, 239,* 586–592.

Ragazzoni, A., Grippo, A., Ghidini, P., Schiavone, V., Lolli, F., Mazzotta, F., et al. (1993). Electrophysiological study of neurologically asymptomatic HIV-1 seropositive patients. *Acta Neurologica Scandinavia, 87,* 47–51.

Rarey, K. E. (1990). Otologic pathophysiology in patients with human immuno-deficiency virus. *American Journal of Otolaryngology, 11,* 366–369.

Real, R., Thomas, M., & Gerwin, J. M. (1987). Sudden hearing loss and acquired immunodeficiency syndrome. *Otolaryngology—Head and Neck Surgery, 97,* 409–412.

Rostad, S. W., Sumi, S. M., Shaw, G. M., Olson, K., & McDougall, J. K. (1987). Human immunodeficiency virus (HIV) infection in brains with AIDS-related leukoencephalopathy. *AIDS Research and Human Retroviruses, 3,* 363–373.

Sahakia, B. J., Elliot, R., Low, N., Mehta, M. Clark, R. T., & Pozmak, A. L. (1995). Neuropsychological deficits in tests of execute function in asymptomatic and symptomatic HIV-1 seropositive men. *Psychological Medicine, 25,* 1233–1246.

Simpson, D. M., & Bender, A. N. (1988). Human immunodeficiency virus-associated myopathy: Analysis of 11 patients. *Annals of Neurology, 24,* 79–84.

Smith, M. E., & Canalis, R. F. (1989). Otologic manifestations of AIDS. The otosyphilis connection. *Laryngoscope, 99,* 365–372.

Sooy, C. D. (1987). Impact of AIDS on otolaryngology-head and neck surgery (vol. 1, pp. 1–28). In E. N. Myers, (Ed.). *Advances in Otolaryngology—Head and Neck Surgery.* Chicago: Year Book Medical Publishers.

Soucek, S., & Michaels, L. (1996). The ear in the acquired immunodeficiency syndrome. II. Clinical and audiologic investigation. *American Journal of Otology, 17,* 35–39.

St. Clair, D. M., Blackwood, D. H. R., & Christie, J. E. (1985). P300 and other long latency auditory evoked potentials in presenile dementia Alzheimer type and alcoholic Korsakoff syndrome. *British Journal of Psychiatry, 147,* 702–706.

Stern, J. C., Lin, P. T., & Lucente, F. E. (1990). Benign nasopharyngeal masses and human Immunodeficiency virus infection. *Archives of Otolaryngology—Head & Neck Surgery, 116,* 206–208.

Syndulko, K., Cohen, S. N., Pettler-Jennings, P., Shah, J., Friedman, A., et al. (1984). P300 and neurocognitive function in neurologic patients (pp. 441–445). In Nodar, P. H., & Barber, C. (Eds.). *Evoked potentials II: The second international evoked potentials symposium, 1984.* Boston: Butterworth.

Timon, C. I., & Walsh, M. A. (1989). Sudden hearing loss as a presentation of HIV infection. *Journal of Laryngology and Otology, 103,* 1071–1072.

Watson, D. W. (1996). Otolaryngologic manifestations of AIDS (pp. 153–158). In Jafek, B. W., Stark, A. K. (Eds). *ENT Secret: Questions you will be asked on rounds, in the clinic, in the O.R., on exams.* Philadelphia: Hanley & Belfus.

Welkoborsky, H., & Lowitzsch, K. (1992). Auditory brain stein responses in patients with immunotropic virus infection of different stages. *Ear and Hearing, 13,* 55–57.

SUGGESTED READINGS

Bergstrom, L., & Thompson, P. L. (1984). Ototoxicity (pp. 119–134). In J. L. Northern, (Ed.), *Hearing disorders.* Austin: Little, Brown.

Chandrasekhar, S. S., Siverls, V., & Sekhar, H. K. (1992). Histopathologic and ultrastructural changes in the temporal bones of HIV-infected human adults. *American Journal of Otology, 13,* 207–214.

Coulman, C. U., Greene, I., & Archibald, R. W. R. (1987). Cutaneous pneumocystosis. *Annals of Internal Medicine, 106,* 396–398.

Eng, R. H., Bishburg, E., Smith, S. M., & Kapila, R. (1986). Cryptococcal infections in patients with acquired immune deficiency syndrome. *American Journal Medicine, 81,* 19–23.

Fallon, J. (1990). Current treatment for human immunodeficiency virus infection. *Ear, Nose and Throat Journal, 69,* 487–496.

Falloon, J., Eddy, J., Wiener, L., & Pizzo, P. A. (1989). Human immunodeficiency virus infection in children. *Journal of Pediatrics, 144,* 1–30.

Linstrom, C. J., & Gleich, L. L. (1993). Otosyphilis: Diagnosis and therapeutic update. *Journal of Otolaryngology, 22,* 401–408.

Lucente, F. E., & Bierstein, K. (1992). Legal, socioeconomic and ethical issues in acquired immunodeficiency syndrome *Otolaryngologic Clinics of North America, 25*(6), 1355–1367.

Mahajan, S. L., Ikeda, Y., & Meyers, T. J. (1981). Acute acoustic nerve palsy associated with vincristine therapy. *Cancer, 47,* 2404–2406.

McArthur, J. C. (1987). Neurologic manifestations of AIDS. *Medicine (Baltimore), 66,* 407–437.

Park, S., Wunderlich, H., Goldenberg, R. A., & Marshall, M. (1992). *Pneumocystis carinii* infection in the middle ear. *Archives of Otolaryngology—Head & Neck Surgery, 118,* 269–270.

Wasserman, L., & Haghighi, P. (1992). Otic and ophthalmic pneumocystosis in acquired immunodeficiency syndrome. *Archives Pathology and Laboratory Medicine, 116,* 500–503.

CHAPTER 4

People with Visual Impairment

Cindy Gustin, PH, MSc
St. Paul's Hospital
Vancouver, British Columbia

Aural Rehabilitation for People with Disabilities

Different senses provide us with different information. Touch offers us opportunities to experience our environment in a somewhat fragmented way, which are limited to objects that are close by and not dangerous. Smell and taste provide only limited information about the world around us, generally require close proximity, and are not always a socially acceptable way to explore an object or person. Vision and hearing are both "distance" senses. They provide us with information about things and events that exist away from our bodies. We rely most heavily on these two senses to learn about the world around us.

Visual impairment has an impact on all aspects of early development, creates challenges with independent living, affects employment opportunities for adults, and increases the risk of isolation for elderly persons. With the absence of vision, access to information from the other intact sensory systems, particularly hearing and touch, is crucial.

Children with visual impairment rely on hearing not only for speech and language development and communication but also for cognitive development and academic success. Visually impaired adults use hearing to access technology that helps them to function independently at home and at work and to participate in leisure activities. Visually impaired individuals of all ages use their hearing to orient themselves to people and things in their environment and to move about safely.

Audiologists rarely receive specific training to assess individuals with visual impairment, and because vision loss is a low-incidence disability, most audiologists have limited opportunity to see these individuals in their practices. It can be intimidating to receive a request to assess someone who is visually impaired or, even worse, suspected of being "deafblind." Nonetheless, early and accurate assessment of hearing is critical to minimize the impact of the sensory impairment(s) and to ensure appropriate management of vision and hearing problems.

The purpose of this chapter is to review the relationship between eye and ear disorders, provide relevant information about visual impairment and its potential impact on audiologic assessment, and present practical suggestions for how to modify audiologic testing to accommodate various visual problems. Interpreting audiologic test results in the context of a visual impairment and providing appropriate recommendations also are discussed.

VISION LOSS: WHAT IT LOOKS LIKE

Vision loss may be due to an eye disorder or brain damage, may be present from birth or acquired later, and may range from partial vision to total blindness. Individuals with vision loss are a heterogeneous population presenting with diverse etiologies, various risk factors, and distinct clinical profiles. Scott, Jan, and Freeman (1995) report that in industrialized nations most children with visual impairment are born with their eye disorders, whereas about one quarter develop their vision loss later in life. Severe visual impairment is uncommon in these countries, occurring in only 6 to 8 children of 10,000. In nonindustrialized nations, childhood blindness is common but is usually acquired. Poor hygiene, malnutrition, vitamin deficiencies, and lack of immunizations predispose children in these countries to infections. It is reported that more than 1 million children develop blindness each year due to devastating eye infections. Most of these children die (Scott et al., 1995).

The National Eye Institute (NEI) reported in 2004 that blindness or low vision affects 3.3 million Americans 40 years or older. By 2020, this figure is projected to reach 5.5 million. The leading causes of visual impairment and blindness in adults in the United States are diabetic retinopathy, age-related macular degeneration, cataracts, and glaucoma (NEI, 2002).

How the Eye Works

The function of the eyes is to focus on an object of interest and then transmit that information to the brain (Scott et al., 1995). A transparent layer called the cornea covers the front of the eye. Light travels through the cornea, passes through the pupil, and continues through the lens. The lens focuses the rays of light on the retina at the back of the eye, which is composed of millions of photoreceptor cells—cones and rods. Near the center of the retina is the macula, a small spot about the size of a pea, which is responsible for processing the fine details of the image. Most cones are located in the macula, whereas most rods are in the periphery of the retina. The macula needs bright light to work well and allows us to see fine detail and color. The remainder of the retina is responsible for peripheral vision, perception of movement, and night vision. At the back of the eye the nerve fibers from the retinal cells come together to form the optic nerve. Messages from the retina travel along the optic nerve to the brain. The visual centers, located in the occipital lobes, receive and then transmit this information to different parts of the brain for analysis (Fig. 4.1).

To see normally, we need eyes that can perceive details up close and at a distance, can distinguish between objects with low contrast, are able to function in various levels of ambient light, and move together in a coordinated fashion. In addition, our brain must be capable of receiving and analyzing the information from the eyes to tell us what we are seeing. It is an undisputed truth that ultimately "we see with our brains rather than our eyes."

Some components of vision, such as visual acuity and peripheral visual fields, can be measured objectively under controlled circumstances. *Legal blindness*, for example, is defined by measurements of visual acuity and/or peripheral visual fields. Visual function is what an individual does with the vision he or she has and may give us a better idea of how some-one manages in their daily life. *Low vision* is more functionally defined as "a visual impairment not correctable by standard glasses, contact lenses, medicine or surgery that interferes with a person's ability to perform everyday activities" (NEI, 2004). Two people may have the same visual acuity but may function differently. In a young child, visual acuity may stay the same but visual function may improve with experience and intervention.

It is critical that clinicians acquire an understanding of the compo-nents of functional vision and the role they play in audiological testing in order to effectively structure the test setting, accurately interpret results, and make appropriate recommendations (Table 4.1).

COMMON EYE DISORDERS

Cataracts

A *cataract* occurs when the normally transparent lens becomes cloudy or opaque. Depending on the size and placement of the cataract, sight may be partially or completely lost until the cataract is removed. Symptoms include cloudy or blurry vision, loss of acuity, difficulty with glare, and poor night vision. *Age-related cataracts*

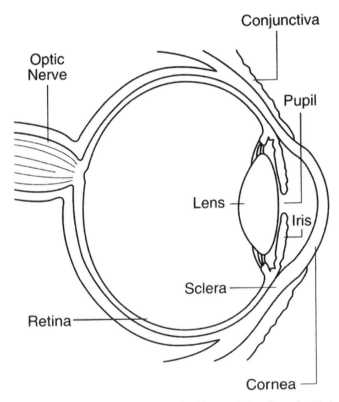

Figure 4.1 Anatomy of the eye. (Reprinted with permission from the National Eye Institute, National Institutes of Health. Reference number NEA05.)

Table 4.1

Components of Functional Vision and Their Potential Impact on Behavioral Audiological Testing

Component	Definition	Normal	Impairment	May impact
Visual acuity	Clarity of vision up close and from a distance. How much an eye sees under controlled circumstances, using 20 feet for distance vision and 16 inches for near vision.	Normal range of vision is 20/20 to 20/70.	May be caused by an unclear lens system, a refractive error, nystagmus (i.e., involuntary eye oscillations), an ocular-motor problem, or damage to retina or optic nerve.	Ability to see and attend to visual reinforcers, to see details of pictures and/or other printed test materials, and to complete some play audiometry tasks. Ability to read written instructions or to access printed material used in counseling. May affect orientation and mobility in test environment.
Visual fields	Areas in which objects are visible without a shift in gaze.	150-degree arcs from right to left and 120-degree arcs up and down.	Reduced visual fields up to and including "tunnel vision." Scotomas (specific areas of vision loss) may vary. *Central visual field loss:* Difficulty seeing detail. *Peripheral visual field loss:* Difficulty detecting movement or locating objects below or to the side may affect mobility. Person may constantly shift position or develop an *eccentric gaze* to compensate.	May appear to have difficulty localizing to sound because of eccentric gaze. May require adjustments to how printed materials and/or objects are displayed. May affect orientation and mobility in test environment.

Oculomotor functioning	Controlled and coordinated movement of eyes.	Eye muscles establish and maintain visual focus, allowing person to scan, fixate, locate, and track objects.	Eye movement disorders may compromise ability to scan horizontally (i.e., oculomotor apraxia). Strabismus compromises focus because direction of eyes is not coordinated.	Ability to efficiently localize or to efficiently scan picture material or objects. Difficulty reading written test instructions and accessing written material used in counseling.
Tolerance for lighting levels	Amount of ambient light required to see.	Daylight or medium artificial illumination is adequate.	Varies according to etiology. Those with retinal disorders require lower lighting, whereas those with myopia or presbyopia may need increased illumination.	Comfort level in the test situation. Ability to see details of pictures or objects or even to function visually in the test environment. May affect orientation and mobility in the test environment.
Contrast sensitivity	Sharpness of contrast required to see things clearly.	Most things in our environment are low contrast. Persons with normal vision do not need the contrast enhanced in order to identify forms.	Inability to see subtle detail (e.g., features of a person's face), given the low contrast between each facial feature and their similarity in color.	Ability to see details of test materials or to read printed materials. May affect orientation and mobility in test environment.

(continued)

Table 4.1

(continued)

Component	Definition	Normal	Impairment	May impact
Cortical vision	Visual centers located in the occipital lobes receive information from the eye and transmit it to various parts of the brain for analysis.	Able to perceive, interpret, and create meaning from the information transmitted by the eye.	Damage to the visual centers or pathways leading to them. Cortical visual impairment can be caused by infection, injury, anoxia, toxins, tumors, or various neurological diseases, and it is frequently associated with additional disabilities. Characterized by visual in-attentiveness; close viewing; prolonged, compulsive light gazing; peripheral field loss; variable visual acuity; and difficulty interpreting visual information. Concurrent eye problems may exist, particularly optic nerve atrophy. Brain damage is common and often severe.	Ability to recognize pictures/objects and to see visual reinforcers. Ability to attend to testing.

Adapted from: Gustin, C. (1997). Audiological Assessment of Children with Visual Impairment. *The Hearing Journal, 50(4)*, 73. (Reprinted with permission from Lippincott Williams & Wilkins.)

are very common in elderly persons, most commonly after age 60 years. *Congenital cataracts* are mostly hereditary but occasionally are caused by a prenatal infection, such as maternal rubella. *Traumatic cataracts,* resulting from an eye injury, can develop at any age. Diabetes mellitus and certain medications also may cause the lens to cloud, creating cataracts.

Glaucoma

Glaucoma is a group of diseases in which increased pressure in the eye causes progressive damage to the retina and optic nerve. Peripheral vision is affected first, and if the condition is untreated, then it can progress to complete blindness. Although commonly associated with aging, glaucoma can affect individuals of any age. It also is common among people who have diabetes. *Congenital glaucoma*, which occurs in children, is usually a genetic condition.

Retinitis Pigmentosa

Retinitis pigmentosa is a heterogeneous group of retinal disorders that can be associated with a number of inherited eye–ear syndromes, most notably Usher's syndrome. The vision loss is caused by degeneration of the retina, and it can affect children or adults. Visual impairment begins with a reduction in peripheral fields, which progresses to tunnel vision and, in some cases, total blindness. In the early stages, individuals with this problem may notice difficulty seeing in dim lighting (night blindness).

Retinopathy of Prematurity

Infants who are born with low birthweight (<1000 g) and are delivered prematurely (26–28 weeks' gestational age) are at risk for developing *retinopathy of prematurity.* Classified in five stages depending on the extent of the damage to the retina, vision loss can range from partial sight to total blindness. Early medical or surgical treatment can now lessen or prevent vision loss. Retinopathy of prematurity may be associated with hearing loss in very low-birthweight infants who survive.

Cytomegalovirus Retinitis

Cytomegalovirus retinitis is a potential complication of AIDS that causes blindness; it occurs in the later stages of the disease when the immune system becomes more severely compromised. It may affect one eye first but usually progresses to both. Symptoms may include scotomas (focal peripheral field loss), blurred vision, and a sudden decrease in vision.

Retinal Detachment

Retinal detachment can occur at any age, but it is most often seen in middle-aged or older people. It can be spontaneous or caused by infection, by injury, and occasionally by heredity. It also can be a complication of diabetes mellitus. Children and adults with severe myopia, such as that seen in Stickler syndrome, may be at risk for retinal detachment. Complete retinal detachment will result in total blindness.

Diabetic Retinopathy

Diabetic retinopathy is a leading cause of blindness in adults; nearly half of all people with diabetes will eventually develop some degree of retinopathy. Changes in the retinal blood vessels affect the macula, causing blurred vision and loss of acuity.

Macular Degeneration

Macular degeneration is the most common cause of blindness in adults in western countries. *Hereditary macular degeneration* occasionally can affect children and adolescents. The most common form is *age-related macular degeneration,* affecting people who are 55 years and older. The severity of the disease can vary, and vision loss may range from mildly distorted or wavy vision, to difficulty reading or performing tasks that require the ability to see fine detail, to complete loss of central vision.

Optic Nerve Atrophy

Optic nerve atrophy can result from various insults to the optic nerve at any age after birth. When the damage to the optic nerve occurs before the end of pregnancy, the optic nerve heads may be small and malformed, resulting in *optic nerve hypoplasia*. Because of advances in medicine, optic nerve atrophy is much less common than it was just a few decades ago.

Corneal Opacity

Corneal opacity is caused by malnutrition and infections. It is the most common type of blindness in the world, but it is seen almost exclusively in underdeveloped countries.

Cortical Visual Impairment

Cortical visual impairment occurs when certain visual areas of the brain have been affected by lack of oxygen, developmental abnormalities, infections, or other diseases or injury. The eyes most often are normal, but acuity still may be severely affected. Variable visual function, visual inattention, light gazing, sensitivity to light, peripheral field loss, and various visual perceptual problems are among the symptoms.

RELATIONSHIP BETWEEN EYE AND EAR DISORDERS

Embryologically, the eye (optic placode) and ear (otic capsule) develop simultaneously from the same type of tissue (neuroectoderm). Any in-utero insult that causes a developmental problem in one system may affect the other (Gustin & Schoem, 1999). Prenatal causes of dual sensory (hearing and visual) impairment can include maternal drug and alcohol abuse; low birthweight related to prematurity and infectious agents, such as cytomegalovirus and herpesvirus; and infections such as toxoplasmosis, acquired immunodeficiency syndrome (AIDS), maternal rubella, and syphilis.

Most inherited hearing loss occurs independently of any other disease process or abnormalities (Jacobsen, 1995). However, in a number of genetic syndromes both hearing and visual impairments are seen. Gustin and Schoem (1999) reported that, of the more than 200 known syndromic hereditary hearing disorders, more than 40 (20%) have associated eye problems. Although recent improvements in prenatal and neonatal care have resulted in a decline in the sporadic (nonhereditary) forms of dual-sensory disorders, an increase in the hereditary types of eye and ear disorders has been seen. Therefore the Joint Committee on Infant Hearing in their Year 2000 Position Statement recommended that "...every infant with hearing loss should receive an ophthalmologic evaluation at regular intervals to rule out late-onset vision disorders" (p. 11).

Acquired hearing or visual impairments may result from infection (e.g., encephalitis, cytomegalovirus, meningitis, AIDS), asphyxia, stroke, or traumatic head injury. Aging also affects both the eye and ear; almost every elderly person experiences some degree of presbycusis (age-related hearing loss), as well as age-related changes in vision (presbyopia) (Table 4.2).

IMPACT OF VISION ON DEVELOPMENT

There is general agreement that vision is probably the most important modality for knowledge acquisition (Lechelt & Hall, 2000). Cognitive, speech and language, motor, and socioemotional development are all affected by vision.

Vision provides immediate and simultaneous access to information about our environment. A child watching a ball roll toward him or her sees the color, shape, and size of the ball as well as how it moves. Using only hearing and touch, a blind child accesses information about the properties and function of a ball in a limited and fragmented way. Vision is also a strong motivator in motor development. The ability to see encourages children to lift their heads, to reach for objects, and to begin to move about in their environment.

A child's speech and language development reflects his or her experience of the world. This differs for sighted and blind children.

Table 4.2

Etiologies of Combined Hearing and Visual Impairment

Etiology	Vision	Hearing
Syndromes/associations/sequences		
Alport syndrome (Type I, II, and VI)	Myopia/cataracts	Progressive sensorineural
Alstrom syndrome	Retinitis pigmentosa	Progressive sensorineural
Cerebral palsy	Optic nerve atrophy/hemianopia	Sensorineural
CHARGE association	Colomboma	Sensorineural and/or conductive
Down's syndrome (Trisomy 21)	Myopia	Sensorineural and/or conductive
Duane syndrome (cervico-oculoacoustic dysplasia)	Eye movement disorder	Sensorineural and/or conductive
Friederich's ataxia	Optic nerve atrophy	Sensorineural
Marshall syndrome	Myopia/cataracts/strabismus	Sensorineural
Neurofibromatosis	Optic nerve atrophy/optic nerve gliomas	Sensorineural
Norrie syndrome (oculoacoustico cerebral degeneration)	Cataract/progressive loss to blindness	Progressive sensorineural
Refsum syndrome	Retinitis pigmentosa	Progressive sensorineural
Stickler's syndrome	Myopia leading to retinal detachment	Sensorineural and/or conductive
Usher syndrome (Types I–III)	Retinitis pigmentosa	Sensorineural
Wolfram syndrome	Optic nerve hypoplasia	Sensorineural
Prenatal		
Infections: congenital rubella, toxoplasmosis, cytomegalovirus (CMV), syphilis, herpes	Optic nerve damage/retinal disorders/cataracts/ cortical visual impairment	Sensorineural
Fetal Alcohol Syndrome (FAS)	Optic nerve damage/cortical visual impairment	Conductive and/or sensorineural
Maternal drug abuse	Optic nerve damage/cortical visual impairment	Sensorineural
Anoxia	Optic nerve hypoplasia/cortical visual impairment	Sensorineural
Prematurity	Retinopathy of prematurity	Sensorineural

(continued)

Table 4.2

(*continued*)

Etiology	Vision	Hearing
Acquired		
Infections: Meningitis/encephalitis/cytomegalovirus, acquired immunodeficiency syndrome (AIDS)	Optic nerve atrophy/cortical visual impairment	Sensorineural
Asphyxia	Optic nerve damage/cortical visual impairment	Sensorineural
Trauma	Optic nerve hypoplasia/cortical visual-impairment/cataracts/retinal bleeding/corneal scarring	Conductive and/or sensorineural
Stroke	Optic nerve hypoplasia/cortical visual impairment	Sensorineural
Aging	Macular degeneration/presbyopia	Sensorineural (presbycusis)

A sighted child's first words usually include names of things that are experienced visually (e.g., "ball", "truck", "doggie"). The early vocabulary of visually impaired children often includes names of objects that have a distinctive feel (e.g., "water"), sound (e.g., "bell"), or smell (e.g., "French fries"). As visually impaired children become older, their vocabulary may reflect more restricted definitions or an imperfect understanding of the properties associated with words. For example, when one of our patients who had been totally blind since birth turned 8 years old, she began insisting that she could now see. When asked for an example of what she could see, she said, "I can see lunchtime."

Vision also plays a pivotal role in the development of auditory skills. Sighted children learn to recognize sounds by hearing a sound, looking to see what made the sound, and putting that information together. Children with visual impairment often need to experience sound (i.e., hold their hand under running water), have it labeled ("water"), and then interpreted ("It's bath time"). A sighted child learns to turn to a sound with the expectation of seeing something. A visually impaired child may stop and listen, turn his or her ear in the direction of a sound, or reach for the sound rather than turning to face the sound source.

The impact of vision loss on an individual depends on a number of factors:

- What are the type and degree of vision loss?
- Is the vision loss congenital or acquired?
- When was the vision loss diagnosed?
- What intervention is provided and when?
- What additional physical, cognitive, and/or sensory impairments are present?

ROLE OF HEARING FOR THE VISUALLY IMPAIRED POPULATION

Human beings hear at several different levels. The *Primitive level* is the most unconscious level of auditory function. Hearing at this level carries the auditory background (sounds that identify the

environment) and the biologic sounds of our bodies (breathing, swallow-
ing, chewing, heartbeat, and pulse). It allows us to feel connected to
our environment and to our own bodies. At the *Signal-Warning/
Passive Learning level*, hearing functions to monitor the world around
us and alert us to danger. It allows us to passively absorb information (including tangential information that is not specifically
directed to us) and social cues. The most sophisticated level of
hearing is the *Symbolic level*, which encompasses active listening and
is responsible for the development of speech and language skills
and spoken communication and for active learning. Individuals
with visual impairment rely more heavily on all levels of hearing
than those with normal vision.

Hearing plays a pivotal role in the development of orientation and
mobility skills. Among the auditory skills described by Hill (1986) as
necessary for orientation and mobility are the following:

- Sound localization
- Sound identification
- Sound discrimination
- Echo location
- Use of sound shadows

Although technology that provides auditory and tactile cues to
assist with independent travel exists, most visually impaired people rely
on echo location. This involves the ability to use sound reflection,
changes in air pressure, the absence of sound, and the identification of
auditory landmarks or changes in auditory background for orientation.
For example, a blind adult needing assistance while shopping may use
the sound of the cash register to locate a staff person.

Auditory aids for the visually impaired include audiotapes, talking
books, talking clocks, talking calculators, and computer applications
that often make use of accelerated, compressed, or synthetic speech.
Efficient use of these technologies depends on good hearing,
effective listening skills, and the ability to retain and process auditory
information.

For the visually impaired, listening is destined to remain a
critical avenue for learning in the classroom. Heinze (1986) lists a
number of skills necessary to effectively learn via hearing, including
the following:

- Basic levels of concentration and attention
- Auditory memory skills
- Fine discrimination of letter sounds
- Vocabulary development
- Auditory closure and the use of context
- Listening for specific purposes
- Selective listening
- Perception of subtle auditory cues that affect meaning, including intonation, intensity, pitch, and pauses

Traditionally audiologists have focused primarily on the symbolic level of hearing when providing an assessment. With the visually impaired population, it is important that we consider all levels of auditory functioning and the auditory needs of each individual.

ASSESSING HEARING IN THE VISUALLY IMPAIRED POPULATION

Vision loss influences how an individual copes in the test environment, how we structure our testing, what test materials we select, what kind of responses we expect to see, how we interpret those responses, and what recommendations we make.

By using information about an individual's visual function to make simple adaptations to the physical setting and test techniques, the clinician's goal is to create a test environment that allows him or her to obtain accurate information about hearing, to interpret test results in the context of the vision loss, and to provide meaningful recommendations. All this should be accomplished with minimal stress to the patient, family, and clinician.

INTERACTING WITH SOMEONE WITH A VISUAL IMPAIRMENT

When meeting and speaking with children and adults who are visually impaired, the clinician should behave in a manner that is sensitive, courteous, and professional. Good manners dictate that the clinician should do the following:

- Speak directly to the visually impaired person, using his or her name.
- Introduce himself or herself and anyone else who may be in the room.
- Do not touch or take hold of the person without warning.
- Speak in a normal manner. Do not avoid words such as "look" or "see" when these words exist as common figures of speech.
- Be sensitive to stereotypes. Not everyone with a visual impairment is a musical prodigy or has developed his or her other senses to paranormal levels.

MOVING ABOUT IN THE TEST ENVIRONMENT

A person with visual impairment may need assistance to move about in the environment. It is important to be sure that the physical setting is as safe as possible. In the test space, special attention should be paid to any potential obstacles such as wires that may be on the floor or boom microphones that can be left pulled out. Be aware that lighting levels can have an impact on vision. Someone who can see well enough to move about easily when the lighting levels are bright may have difficulty seeing in the dimmer light of a sound booth.

When the client moves from one area to another, ask if "guided assistance" is needed. If assistance is required, then offer your arm. An adult will grasp your elbow whereas a child may hold onto your wrist. This position allows you to remain beside and slightly ahead as you walk. Doors should be fully open or closed to avoid accidents. As you move through a doorway, describe where you are going. You may assist the person to grasp the door to clear it. Verbally identify any obstacles, such as steps up or down into the booth or wires on the floor. When you guide the person to a chair, place his or her hand on the back of the chair, tell the person that it is a chair, and that you would like him or her to sit down. Make sure that the person is aware of any other objects, such as a boom microphone or table, which may be in the vicinity. If possible, ensure that obstacles are removed. In addition to physical guidance, a running commentary orienting the visually impaired person to what the physical space is like, where you are going, and what you are doing is helpful.

If guided assistance is declined, then it is appropriate to provide verbal guidance. Describe the physical space and the location of furniture or other objects. When identifying furniture, you may want to give a sound cue as well, such as tapping a table, to help the person locate it. A cloth of contrasting color on the back of a chair or reflective tape on a threshold or step can make it easier to see.

Warn the person before touching him or her. Do not assume that the person will see you approach. Before using an otoscope or placing a headset or insert phones, describe what you are about to do. With adults you may only need to describe the phones or headsets. With children, you may wish to let them explore the piece of equipment before using it. When you use a boom microphone for speech testing, caution the visually impaired person that the microphone will be placed in front of him or her and allow the person to locate the position of the microphone by touch if necessary. Again, it is important to provide a verbal commentary for each step of the assessment.

TESTING ADULTS WITH VISUAL IMPAIRMENT

Visually impaired adults are usually able to provide standard, unambiguous responses to pure tone and speech testing so that adaptations of the audiologic test battery are not necessary. Adaptations for testing adults with a visual impairment generally involve obtaining information about the type and degree of vision loss (case history), modifying the physical environment, and ensuring accessibility to any printed materials.

CASE HISTORY

A question about the status of vision should always be included in a case history, even if no vision loss is suspected. This question can be as simple as asking whether the person is aware of any problems with the eyes or vision. If a visual impairment is reported, then information about the cause of the vision loss, specifically how vision is affected and under what circumstances the person has difficulty seeing, will be important to set up the test environment, to interpret the results, and to make appropriate recommendations.

LIGHTING

Simply put, the most common problem with lighting is that it is either too bright, resulting in a glare, or is not bright enough. Lighting in the test setting should be as flexible as possible. A dimmer switch that allows lighting levels in the sound booth to be adjusted can be helpful. Lighting should be task specific. Table lamps can be placed to provide optimal lighting. A penlight or flashlight can be used if more light is needed for reading printed materials. Minimizing the use of reflective or highly polished surfaces or covering them with cloth will help reduce glare.

PRINTED MATERIALS

Printed test materials, test instructions, and counseling information should be made available in large print. A font size of 16 point is recommended, and a sans serif font, such as Arial or Universal, is easier to read. Both capital and small letters should be used. Printing should be on a plain background, on one side of the paper only, and should be spaced to avoid crowding.

Laminating or placing printed material in a plastic page protector may cause glare. Printed materials can be mounted instead on lightweight cardboard to increase durability and to ensure that light does not penetrate the paper when it is held up to read. A handheld magnifier, which may come with a light attachment, can be used with any printed materials. If a test involves choosing from a set of written responses, then the printed material should be easy to hold or to move close to the visually impaired person's face when necessary. For example, printed material mounted on cardboard may be lighter and easier to hold up than papers attached to a clipboard. A slant board with a clip to hold printed material, which can be placed on a table in front of the person being tested, may be another option.

TESTING CHILDREN WITH VISUAL IMPAIRMENT

Audiologic testing of visually impaired children presents audiologists with a unique set of challenges. First, standard pediatric test techniques involve a large component of functional vision. This is true not only for Visual Reinforcement Audiometry but also for Behavioral Observation and Conditioned Play Audiometry (Gustin, 1997). Second, children with visual impairments frequently present with additional disabilities. A review of the literature by Lechelt and Hall (2000) indicated that "the frequency of disabilities additional to blindness is so high that a sample of children with no additional disabilities other than congenital blindness might not represent the general population of children who are congenitally blind" (p. 2). Disabilities include developmental delay, brain injury, autism, and physical disabilities such as cerebral palsy. Typically any one of these disabilities would place the child in the "difficult to test" category. Finally, vision loss is a low-incidence disability. Audiologists in general practice rarely see these children, making it difficult to gain experience and develop expertise with this population.

Ideally audiologic testing of children with visual impairment should be done as part of a multidisciplinary assessment, particularly if the diagnosis of vision loss is new. Just as it is unrealistic to expect audiologists to have specific training or experience in the area of visual impairment, professionals with expertise related to low vision or blindness generally lack training and experience in the area of hearing impairment. In addition, children with a dual sensory impairment (i.e., deafblind) present with different needs than either visually impaired or hearing impaired children and require unique management. A team approach allows professionals and families to coordinate information and share expertise (Gustin, 1997).

Early detection of hearing loss is important both diagnostically and for implementing treatment. Normal hearing should also be confirmed as soon as possible to provide appropriate counseling in the context of the vision loss. In our clinic, once a visual impairment is confirmed or when the child is known to have a condition involving vision loss, hearing testing is among the first assessments to be scheduled.

MAKING THE CHILD MORE TESTABLE

Traditionally, one method of assessing children who are considered difficult to test is to have them return over several sessions for serial audiograms. Although this can be effective, it can also be costly and time consuming for families, children, and clinicians. If the family must travel long distances to the audiology clinic, it may not be feasible. One alternative is to provide the parents or school with a mediator-based conditioning program that teaches the child a consistent behavioral response to sound. These responses can then be generalized to formal behavioral audiologic testing. The advantage of this option is that the children come to their assessment already familiar with what they must do during testing and the parents arrive with a wealth of infor-mation about what responses to expect, what sounds elicit the best responses, what is most reinforcing to the child, and what does not work (Gustin, 1997).

TEST BATTERY

As with sighted children, children with visual impairment are assessed using a battery of tests. Each test must be interpreted in light of the other tests. Test results should make sense and should not contradict each other.

The test battery may include both objective and subjective tests. For populations that are considered difficult to test, it is tempting to rely heavily on physiologic tests, such as Auditory Brainstem Response and Otoacoustic Emissions testing. The importance of normal hearing in both ears for sound localization and the advantage of binaural hearing in noisy situations, particularly when there is limited access to visual cues to supplement hearing, means that for children with vision loss, indivi-dual ear thresholds should be determined as soon as possible. Physiologic tests are helpful to obtain this information in very young visually impaired children or those with additional disabilities. Confirmation of behavioral findings by objective measures can also be reassuring to parents and also to the clinician.

When previous audiologic testing has been unsuccessful, there is the danger that undue emphasis can be placed on the physiologic tests. By definition, these tests indicate "a patient's hearing ability without the patient's active participation in the test" and do not reflect hearing in the sense of "meaningful interpretation of the sound as to produce thought and language" (Northern & Downs, 2002). Although we recognize the importance of these tests as part of the test battery, it is our conviction that accurate behavioral testing provides us with the richest information about how a child hears and uses that hearing.

CASE HISTORY

For children, questions should cover standard pediatric case history information, information related to additional disabilities that may have an impact on the testing and information about functional vision and hearing. Often information about a child's formal visual diagnosis, visual acuity measurements, peripheral visual field defects, or sensitivity to light is not available before audiologic testing. This sort of information can be elicited by asking the following questions:

- How well does your child see?
- Can your child see your face?
- Can your child see you from across the room?
- Does your child see better on one side or the other?
- Does your child see better in dim light or bright light?
- Does your child like lights?
- Will your child stare at lights?
- Do bright lights bother your child?
- Does your child look directly at what he or she is trying to see?
- Does your child tilt his or her head when he or she is looking at something?
- Can you get your child to look at something by using sound?
- Do your child's eyes shake?

Most parents can provide a great deal of information about their child's functional vision. If you know which questions to ask, then you will find that parents usually know the answers.

ADAPTING BEHAVIORAL TESTING

Adaptations of behavioral testing to accommodate visual impairment are divided here into low-technology and high-technology categories. Low-technology suggestions include adaptations that can be made with little expense, using household items or versions of audiologic test materials that are commercially available. They can often be made on the spot or with a little advanced planning. This category would probably be most useful to those clinicians who see children with visual impairment only occasionally in their practices. High-technology options may involve greater expense, customized equipment, and/or equipment that is not typically used in audiologic testing. This may be useful to clinicians who see a number of children with visual impairment regularly. We have found these modifications to be useful with sighted children and with children who are cognitively or physically challenged as well.

Adapting the Physical Environment

Adaptations to the physical environment typically come down to lighting and background.

As with adults, the ability to adjust lighting levels in the test environment can make a significant difference in a child's comfort level and ability to perform during testing. Not all visually impaired children do better in bright light. Some patients with retinal disorders, for example, do better in dim light. Similarly, those with normal acuity do not require a lot of contrast to see, whereas others with visual impairment do. When pictures or objects are displayed during testing, backgrounds should be plain and should offer good contrast. It is important to be aware of potential problems with glare from lighting sources or reflective surfaces.

The following are some low-technology adaptations:

- A pair of children's sunglasses can be used if lighting levels are uncomfortably bright (Fig. 4.2).
- A hat with a brim, such as a baseball cap, can shade the eyes from overhead lighting.
- A desk lamp can provide increased or task-specific lighting.
- Plain, solid-colored felt, cork, or Dycem boards are best for displaying objects or materials. Dycem is particularly useful for displaying pictures, because it will help hold them in place.
- Plain, solid-colored tablecloths can be used to cover tables or "see-through" (clear) wheelchair trays, providing a solid color background for improved contrast and reduction in potential glare.

The following are some high-technology adaptations:

- Dimmer switches on overhead lights in the booth allow for flexibility in lighting levels.
- Commercially available light boxes with adjustable lighting levels offer greater contrast for displaying test materials and objects.

Adapting the Test Materials

The selection of test materials (familiar objects, picture cards, and play audiometry materials) and how they are presented or displayed may need to be modified. We must consider how much vision is involved in each activity. Tasks that can be performed more easily by touch or tasks for which touch can supplement vision to make them easier or more interesting will probably work best.

The following are low-technology adaptations:

- Select games that require less vision or that can easily be accomplished by touch, such as stacking cups or dropping blocks in a bucket. A tactile board with circular pieces of differing textures that fit into spots on the board may be a more interesting play task for a child with limited vision.

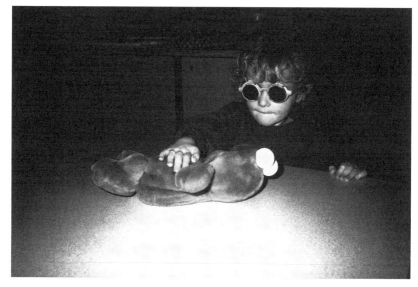

Figure 4.2 Sunglasses can be used to adjust lighting levels in the test environment and thereby increase a child's comfort level and ability to perform during testing. Toys that produce an auditory or tactile response can be very reinforcing for children who have low vision or blindness. (Photo printed with permission.)

- Building towers of pegs may be easier and more interesting for a child with low vision than use of a traditional pegboard (Fig. 4.3).
- Have the family bring a familiar picture book from home that the child is able to see. An informal speech reception threshold can be obtained by having the child point to pictures in the book.
- Use of individual picture cards of familiar objects or spondee items, such as those from the Picture Spondee Threshold Test, allows the clinician to preferentially select items that the child knows, have good contrast, and can be easily seen (Fig. 4.4). Individual cards can be displayed in ways to accommodate visual crowding, visual field losses, or eye movement disorders that affect a child's ability to visually scan.
- Body part identification or familiar objects can be used if pictures are too difficult for the child to see. Be careful when selecting familiar objects to use with children who are blind or severely visually impaired. To a young, blind child, taste, texture, and temperature are among the properties that allow them to identify items such as "ice cream" or "popcorn." Plastic representations of these, which can be used to assess sighted children, may not be appropriate for a visually impaired child. Real-life items, such as "toothbrush" or "baseball" may be better choices.
- A slant board for displaying picture materials may make pictures more visually accessible for some children.

The following are high-technology adaptations:

- Commercially available light boxes can be used to display familiar objects or pictures. Some familiar object cards that are available for purchase with the light boxes are, in fact, spondee items.
- A light box with colored pegs and a grid may be easier to use visually or by touch than a traditional pegboard, and the task is more interesting than dropping blocks in a bucket (Fig. 4.5).

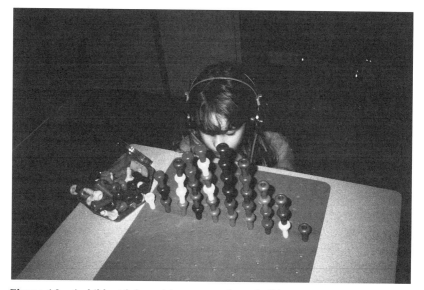

Figure 4.3   A child with low vision may prefer to build a tower of pegs rather than use a traditional pegboard, because creating a tower may be easier to do by touch and more interesting for the child. (Photo printed with permission.)

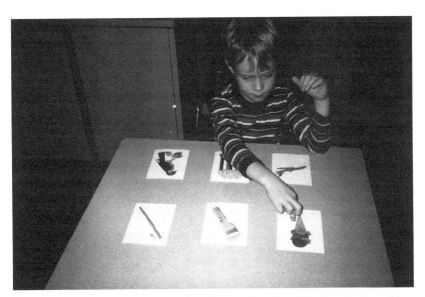

Figure 4.4   Individual Picture Spondee Cards can be selected for familiarity and best visual contrast, and can then be displayed to avoid visual crowding and to allow for ease of visual scanning. (Photo printed with permission.)

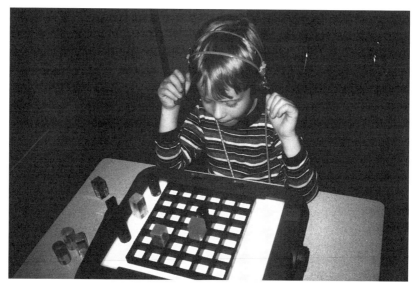

Figure 4.5   A grid and colored pegs on a light box may make a play audiometry task easier for a child with low vision and may encourage attention to task. (Photo printed with permission.)

Adapting Reinforcers

Much of what is reinforcing about pediatric testing comes from vision. Most visually impaired children do have useful sight and may be able to access visual reinforcers. Social reinforcement can also be very effective with visually impaired children. However, be aware that nonverbal social reinforcement, such as smiling, nodding, and using thumbs-up signs, may not be visually accessible to them. We need to ask ourselves: What is reinforcing about this task? How much of that is visual? Does this child have enough vision to access this reinforcement? Can reinforcement come from another sense, such as touch? How can I make the reinforcement more accessible to the child?

Visual Reinforcement Audiometry

The following are low-technology adaptations:

- Visual reinforcers with animation and lights are more versatile than those with lights only.
- Visual reinforcers that can be moved about the sound booth can accommodate a number of visual defects.
- Removable front panels on shadow boxes allow for easier visibility.

The following are high-technology adaptations:

- Customized visual reinforcement audiometry (VRA) system. Our VRA system uses three sets of animated toys, mounted on two stands that can be adjusted for distance and height or removed completely from the stands and placed next to the child. This allows us to accommodate for acuity problems, visual field defects, and physical limitations (i.e., limited head and neck mobility). The toys can be set for lights and animation or lights only, and the shadow boxes can be opened to allow better access to the reinforcers (Fig. 4.6).

Conditioned Play Audiometry

The following are low-technology adaptations:

- Chose objects with various shapes and textures for some version of the traditional "blocks in a bucket" task.

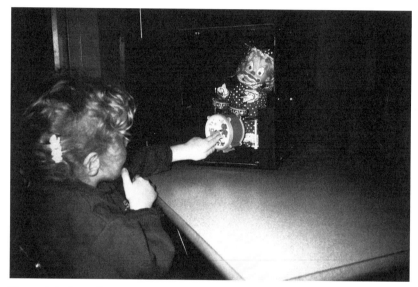

Figure 4.6   Sets of animated toys mounted in movable shadow boxes with removable covers allow for better visual and tactile access to reinforcers. (Photo printed with permission.)

- Interconnecting pegs or stacking cups may be more interesting and possibly easier to use by touch if there is a severe visual impairment.
- Animated toys removed from their shadow boxes can be used to provide tactile reinforcement.
- Older children can earn tokens that can be used to buy a prize at the end of testing.

The following are high-technology adaptations:

- A light box with a grid and colored pegs may be more accessible visually or by touch.
- A "flashing stamp" that lights up when it is pressed may be a more interesting task for someone with low vision. For children who can see well enough, a paper with circles or a path or some other pattern can be filled with stamps.
- A Tickle Me Elmo or similar toy that gives auditory and tactile reinforcement when the child touches it in response to a stimulus can be very motivating. We caution that these should be only used with children who are reliable responders because it can be difficult to control for false-positive responses.

INTERPRETING RESPONSES

The goal of modifying our test techniques and materials is to create an environment that allows the child to give an unambiguous response to the auditory stimuli. As long as responses are clear and consistent, they are adequate for testing purposes. Clinicians must assess the child's baseline state and decide which responses are acceptable. Flexibility in following the child's lead is essential.

Behavioral responses should be interpreted beyond simply presence versus absence. The type, quality, and variety of responses provide important information about what a child hears and how he or she uses that information. It is our practice to record the specific behaviors we observed and considered to be responses, which stimuli elicited the best responses, and how we modified our testing to obtain this information (Gustin & Schoem, 1999).

Once all the appropriate modifications have been made, responses must be interpreted in the context of the specific vision loss. A young, blind child may reach for a sound rather than turn his or her head or may turn his or her "ear" toward the sound rather than turning to face the sound source, appearing to localize in the wrong direction. A child with damaged maculas and central vision may develop an "eccentric gaze," that is, may fixate above, below, or to the side of the object of interest to see it. Nystagmus may increase if a child is tired, anxious, or trying hard to see. An increase in eye oscillations after an auditory stimulus may mean the child is trying to look for what made the sound and, under certain circumstances, could be interpreted as a behavioral response to sound.

We need to be aware that children with visual impairment may take longer to respond during testing. A child with low vision may need extra time to focus on an object or to scan printed materials. Nystagmus can make it more difficult for a child to read. If responses require extended effort on the part of the child to use vision, then fatigue may become a factor. Additional disabilities may also interfere with the child's ability to give a clear and rapid response to sound.

MANAGEMENT

Audiologic findings should be interpreted, and subsequent recommendations made in the context of the vision loss. In the presence of a visual impairment, findings of either normal hearing or hearing impairment have implications for the following:

- Development of speech and language, cognitive, motor, and socioemotional abilities
- Communication
- Academic success
- Employment opportunities
- Orientation and mobility
- Access to technology for the visually impaired
- Therapies that promote the use of vision
- Safety skills
- Quality of life

Depending on the results of audiologic testing, individuals can generally be placed into one of three categories: those who are visually impaired but have normal hearing, those with some degree of coexisting visual and hearing impairment, and those who are considered to be deafblind. Management options vary for each group.

Visual Impairment with Normal Hearing

For visually impaired children and adults who have normal hearing, management is generally limited to providing information about the interaction of vision and hearing. Information will vary, depending on the person's age; the type, degree, and onset of vision loss; the presence of any additional disabilities; and the specific needs or lifestyle choices of each individual.

Counseling topics may include, but are not limited to, the following:

- Causes of transient hearing loss and their impact on someone with a visual impairment. Patients and families should be cautioned that temporary or fluctuating hearing loss related to upper respiratory tract infections or excessive cerumen is more significant for those who are visually impaired. Prompt medical treatment is recommended to ensure that hearing remains as good as possible.

- Explicit recommendations about hearing conservation, both for children and adults. The potential effects of ototoxic medications and noise exposure and the use of hearing protection when appropriate should be discussed.

- Communicating under difficult listening conditions. Situations in which there is background noise, in which the speaker has a soft voice or is speaking at a distance, or in which the speaker cannot be seen are considered difficult listening conditions. Sighted people use visual cues to supplement their hearing in these situations. Depending on the environment, the amount of residual vision, and the visually impaired person's ability to use this vision, his or her ability to access compensatory visual information may be limited. Awareness of what constitutes a difficult listening situation and ways of compensating under these conditions (i.e., reducing background noise or moving away from its source, moving closer to the speaker, or adjusting position or lighting to maximize access to visual cues) should be discussed.

For children, some additional information should be provided, including the following:

- The impact of vision loss on normal auditory development. Children who can hear sounds that originate outside their visual range may need to be specifically taught which of these sounds are important to them and what they mean. Parents should be counseled that their child's responses to sound might be different from those of sighted children. For example, their child may not turn to face sounds but may be still and listen or reach for the sound instead.
- The potential impact of visual impairment on the development of receptive and expressive language skills. Children with good hearing and good auditory memory may remember and use words that they do not fully understand. These children may appear to be fluent talkers, but comprehension skills may lag behind expressive language skills. Parents should be alerted to this fact so that speech and language development can be monitored and intervention arranged if necessary.
- A child with a visual impairment may be a visual learner. Although we may counsel that hearing is adequate for the academic needs of this group of children, we should not assume that they are, in fact, auditory learners. A visually impaired child may be a visual learner. Parents should be advised to carefully monitor academic progress.
- Routine monitoring of hearing is recommended even if no hearing loss has been diagnosed. For visually impaired children, audiologic assessment is recommended at least once a year. Hearing may be monitored more often for specific children depending on risk factors, age, status of visual impairment, and the child's ability to indicate whether he or she is having any difficulty hearing. Adults with vision loss should also have

their hearing assessed periodically. Hearing may be monitored less often for adults, because they will be able to request testing if they notice changes in their hearing.

VISUAL IMPAIRMENT AND HEARING IMPAIRMENT

Clinically, for individuals presenting with concurrent vision and hearing problems, one sensory system is usually deemed to be more significantly affected than the other. For example, an individual may be treated as a hearing impaired person who does not see too well or as a visually impaired person who has some difficulty hearing. It is assumed that one sense is at least partially able to compensate for the other. If audiologic testing confirms a hearing loss, then the combined effect of these impairments must be considered. Management will vary depending on the clinical profile.

Counseling topics may include, but are not be limited to, the following:

- The consideration of any degree of hearing loss as significant when there is a concomitant vision loss.
- The greater impact of mild, fluctuating, or transient hearing loss for visually impaired people who have limited ability to supplement their hearing with visual cues.
- The impact of hearing loss on all levels of auditory function. For example, a unilateral hearing loss should not significantly interfere with speech and language development but can interfere with hearing in difficult listening situations and can have an impact on the ability to localize sound, affecting orientation and mobility, and personal safety for a person with a vision loss.
- The potential impact of the hearing loss on a child's ability to access auditory cues during therapy to promote the use of vision or an adult's ability to access technology for the visually impaired.
- Management of hearing loss with medical or surgical treatment or amplification. Hearing loss should be managed more aggressively, either with medical or surgical treatment when appropriate or with amplification when there is a coexisting visual impairment.

- The person's ability to use residual vision to compensate for the hearing loss or residual hearing for the vision loss. For example, is the person able to see detail well enough to lip-read, see facial expressions, or access other visual information to supplement hearing? Awareness of situations in which the person may have difficulty seeing or hearing and ways in which he or she can maximize residual vision or hearing should be discussed.

- Team approach to management. Support personnel for individual sensory impairments, such as a teacher of the deaf and hard of hearing and a teacher of the visually impaired, should be in close contact and work together to ensure that recommendations are consistent and services are administered efficiently.

- Early intervention. If the underlying etiology indicates a progressive hearing and/or visual impairment, then supports should be put in place early. For example, lip-reading and/or sign language can be taught while the person still has residual hearing. If the dual sensory impairment is expected to progress to deafblindness, then cochlear implantation may be performed while the person still has enough vision to support the adjustment to the sound from a cochlear implant and the development of speech understanding.

- Choice of manual communication. If sign language is recommended, either because of the degree of hearing loss or because of an additional disability that affects speech, then the type and degree of vision loss may affect the choice of sign language. Eye disorders that affect the ability to see fine detail, reduce visual fields, or create scotomas may make it difficult for the individual to access some signs. For example, the American Sign Language sign for "go" is easier to see than the sign for the same word in Signed Exact English.

DEAFBLIND

Individuals who are considered to be *deafblind* or *dual sensory impaired* are a unique group requiring unique management. People who are deafblind may experience the world in a fragmented or limited way.

For these individuals, the world may seem unpredictable or even threatening (Miles, 2000).

Definitions of deafblindness vary, but criteria usually include (1) a combination of visual impairment and hearing impairment that creates difficulty in communication, mobility, concept development, access to information, development of independence in daily life activities, psychosocial adjustment, and obtaining a vocation, and where (2) these deficits create unique needs requiring specialized services and modified educational programs beyond those provided for individuals who are deaf or blind or multiply handicapped (Arizona Deafblind Project, 2002).

Very few people who are classified as deafblind are completely without sight or hearing. Most have some residual vision or hearing. Often, additional disabilities are present in this population. It has been reported that as many as 80% of children identified as deafblind have additional disabling conditions, including cognitive impairment, physical handicaps, and social or emotional problems (Arizona Deafblind Project, 2002; Miles, 2000). Because deafblindness is a combination of vision and hearing loss, there is no single profile for someone who is deafblind and, therefore, no single method of managing this condition.

The impact of deafblindness will depend on a number of factors, including age of onset, degree and type of vision and hearing loss, stability of each sensory loss, and intervention provided (Arizona Deafblind Project, 2002). Audiologic management for this population may include many of the recommendations listed in the previous section. Our goal is to optimize residual hearing with referrals for medical or surgical assessments and by fitting amplification, and to provide useful information about the interaction of the hearing loss and vision loss for each individual.

Early and direct intervention by professionals who are trained in the field of deafblindness, in programs specifically designed to meet the unique needs of these individuals, is required to minimize the impact of the coexisting visual and hearing problems. Because of the diversity of needs, services can rarely be provided by a single person or agency (Miles, 2000). Management of both children and adults is best provided in the context of a team approach, involving families, professionals, and agencies.

REFERENCES

Arizona Deafblind Project. (2002). *What is deafblindness?* Retrieved from http://www.azdb.org/whatsdb.1htm.

Gustin, C. (1997). Audiological testing of children with a visual impairment. *The Hearing Journal, 50*(4), 70–75.

Gustin, C., & Schoem, S. R. (1999). Testing hearing in children who are visually impaired: Why, when and how. Paper presented at Here's Lookin' at You, Kid2: The Ninth International Conference on Blind and Visually Impaired Children, Calgary, Alberta, Canada.

Heinze, T. (1986). Communication skills (pp. 304–314). In Scholl, G. T. (Ed.). *Foundations of education for blind and visually handicapped children and youth: Theory and practice.* New York: American Foundation for the Blind.

Hill, E. W. (1986). Orientation and mobility. In Scholl, G. T. (Ed.). *Foundations of education for blind and visually handicapped children and youth: Theory and practice.* New York: American Foundation for the Blind.

Jacobson, J. T. (1995). Nosology of deafness. *Journal of American Academy of Audiology, 6,* 15–20.

Joint Committee on Infant Hearing. (2000, August). Year 2000 Position Statement: Principals and guidelines for early hearing detection and intervention programs [Special Issue]. *Audiology Today.*

Lechelt, E. C., & Hall, D. L. (2000). *The impact of vision loss on the development of children from birth to 12 years: A literature review.* Retrieved from The Canadian National Institute for the Blind Web site:http://www.cnib.ca/eng/fps/vision.loss/index.htm.

Miles, B. (2000). *Overview on deaf-blindness.* Retrieved from DB-Link: National Information Clearinghouse on Children Who Are Deaf-Blind Web site: http://www.tr.wou.edu/dblink/overview.htm.

National Eye Institute. (2001). *Anatomy of the eye.* National Institutes of Health. Reference number NEA05. Retrieved from http://www.nei.nih.gov.

National Eye Institute. (2004). National Eye Health Education Program (NEHEP). *Frequently asked questions about low vision.* Retrieved from http://www.nei.nih.gov/nehep/faqs.asp.

National Eye Institute. (2004). Prevalence and causes of visual impairment and blindness among adults 40 years and older in the United States. *Vision loss from eye diseases will increase as Americans age.* Retrieved from http://www.nei.nih.gov/news/pressreleases/041204.asp.

Northern, J. L., & Downs, M. P. (2002). *Hearing in children* (5th ed.). New York: Lippincott, Williams & Wilkins.

Scott, E. P., Jan, J. E., & Freeman, R. D. (1995). *Can't your child see? A guide for parents and professionals about young children who are visually impaired* (3rd ed.). Austin, TX: PRO-ED.

CHAPTER 5

Older Adults with Dementia or Alzheimer's Disease

Emi Isaki, Ph.D., CCC/SLP
Division of Speech Pathology and Audiology
John A. Burns School of Medicine
University of Hawaii at Manoa
Honolulu, HA

Prevalence of Dementia

Hearing Loss in the Normal Elderly Population

Hearing Loss and Cognitive Dysfunction

Ethics of Service Provision

Identification and Evaluation of Dementia

Management

Summary

Acknowledgments

References

This chapter reviews how changes in cognition, communication, behavior, and emotion associated with dementia or Alzheimer's disease (AD) can affect the provision of audiologic services. The problems associated with hearing loss in the normal aging population can also exist in individuals with dementia or AD. However, the progressive decline of cognitive and communicative abilities in an individual with dementia or AD can make the identification of an actual hearing loss more difficult, especially as the disease progresses into the moderate or middle stages. Therefore during audiologic evaluation and aural rehabilitation, a team approach involving the client, family members, caregivers, and health care professionals is needed to ensure accurate assessment, carry out recommendations, and provide the best care possible.

PREVALENCE OF DEMENTIA

Dementia generally occurs in the elderly population. Approximately 5–8% of individuals older than age 65 years have some form of dementia with the incidence doubling every 5 years ("Dementia," 2003). Of the various types of dementia, AD is the most common, affecting approximately 4 million people in the United States (Alzheimer's Association, 2004).

Dementia is a broad medical term used to describe different types of gradually progressive degenerative diseases affecting the brain. Dementia is often initially identified by the individual or family members and diagnosed by physicians and neuropsychologists. The *Diagnostic and Statistical Manual of Mental Disorders* (American Psychiatric Association, 1994) describes various types of dementia with specific inclusionary and exclusionary criteria for diagnoses. For instance, an example of an inclusionary criterion for a diagnosis of dementia of the Alzheimer's type is that the client displays multiple cognitive deficits with progressive decline in areas such as memory and executive functions that affect social interaction or employment (*DSM-IV*). An example of an exclusionary criterion for this diagnosis would be that the cognitive deficits are not attributable to other central nervous system conditions such as cerebrovascular accidents (i.e., stroke) or systemic conditions (*DSM-IV*).

Recent advancements in the early detection of dementia and increased awareness by the general population have caused the number of individuals identified with the disease to rise. For instance, an estimated 7 million individuals in the United States have some form of mild to severe dementia ("Dementia," 2003). The Alzheimer's Association (2004) estimates that by the year 2050, 14 million Americans will have AD. Therefore unless effective medical management or treatment is found, the number of individuals with the diagnosis of dementia will certainly continue to increase.

HEARING LOSS IN THE NORMAL ELDERLY POPULATION

The National Institute on Aging (2002) reported that approximately one third of Americans older than age 60 years have some type of hearing problem, and the incidence increases to about one half of the U.S. population for individuals older than age 85 years. Hearing loss in elderly persons may be attributed to various causes such as normal aging, excess cerumen, noise exposure, medications, infections, injuries, or genetics (National Institute on Aging, 2002). Presbycusis, or high-frequency hearing loss, is a common occurrence that has been well documented in individuals as they age. Weinstein (2000) defines presbycusis as a chronic health-related condition described as hearing loss associated with aging, which presents as an insidious, progressive, high-frequency, sensorineural hearing impairment.[*] Thus individuals who have presbycusis mainly have problems hearing high-frequency speech sounds, which can affect communication. Therefore individuals with this type of hearing loss may have difficulty understanding normal conversation, especially in noisy environments. To enhance communication abilities and increase quality of life, an audiologist will routinely prescribe a hearing aid or aids or assistive listening devices and assist in aural rehabilitation.

Another common occurrence that affects hearing in the elderly population is an accumulation of cerumen (earwax). The buildup of earwax can cause a conductive hearing loss in older individuals. After removal of the cerumen, either hearing may be restored or the severity of the hearing loss may be lessened (Allen et al., 2003). The National Institute on Aging (2002) stated that in addition to excess cerumen, a conductive hearing loss can also result from middle ear fluid buildup, abnormal bone growth, a punctured eardrum, or middle ear infection.

Finally, tinnitus is present in the elderly population. Tinnitus is typically described as ringing in the ears and can coexist with hearing loss. Tinnitus can occur from exposure to loud noise, hearing loss, medications, or health problems such as allergies (National Institute on Aging, 2002). External noise that masks the tinnitus can be used to lessen the problem.

In general, when an individual has concerns about a hearing problem, a formal evaluation is recommended. This evaluation can involve health care professionals such as an otolaryngologist and an audiologist (National Institute on Aging, 2002). After the hearing evaluation, suggestions can be made such as the use of a hearing aid or aids for presbycusis or the removal of excess cerumen for improved hearing. Therefore

---

[*]From Weinstein, B. E. (2000). *Geriatric audiology.* New York: Thieme Medical Publishers. Reprinted by permission.

acquiring services from health care professionals who are knowledgeable in hearing function and remediation will be extremely valuable to the individual with a hearing loss.

HEARING LOSS AND COGNITIVE DYSFUNCTION

Commonly occurring problems such as presbycusis and excessive cerumen that influence normal hearing in elderly individuals are also evident in individuals with dementia. Thus sensorineural hearing loss, conductive hearing loss, and tinnitus can also occur in this population. In addition to the problems associated with normal aging, individuals with dementia or AD have other obstacles that can influence hearing ability. Progressive changes in cognition in the areas of attention or working (short-term) memory can affect communication abilities such as receptive language skills (Hopper, Bayles, & Kim, 2001). In turn, these problems can make the audiologic assessment and aural rehabilitation process difficult for individuals with dementia and the health care professionals working with them.

Individuals with dementia or AD begin to lose cognitive abilities progressively over time. Cognition or skills that assist one in thinking help individuals to function in everyday life. Cognitive skills are necessary for daily activities, work, education, and obtaining new information or skills (Brookshire, 2003). Areas of cognition that can become impaired with dementia or AD include attention, memory, organization, problem solving, reasoning, judgment, and executive functions (Brookshire, 2003). Specific cognitive skills such as selective or divided attention and memory for events and new learning, which influence communication, begin to deteriorate early in the progression of the disease (Hopper et al., 2001).

In addition to reduced cognitive skills, a related problem that can affect an individual with dementia or AD is depression. Depression may occur if the client recognizes changes in his or her everyday thinking abilities. Brookshire (2003) stated that symptoms of depression could often be mistaken for symptoms of dementia. Thus depression may influence cognitive processes negatively, oftentimes producing a pseudodementia (Brookshire, 2003). The pseudodementia can produce characteristics similar to those of dementia with problems evident in memory, attention, and orientation (Brookshire, 2003).[*] However, if depression occurs in conjunction with dementia or AD, cognitive deficits can appear to be more severely affected than those in an individual without depression. Therefore if family members, caregivers, health care professionals, or the client with dementia notice any signs of depression, the client should be referred for appropriate services. The treatment of depression may positively influence how an individual with dementia performs on cognitively demanding tasks and in his or her daily routines. Therefore addressing the depression before an audiologic evaluation and aural rehabilitation is imperative for an individual with dementia or AD if one expects him or her to perform to the best of his or her abilities.

Schow and Nerbonne (2002) reported that audiologists assume the major role in providing education and instruction about aural rehabilitation to clients. However, other disciplines are often involved in the aural rehabilitation process. These professionals can include psychologists, social workers, rehabilitation counselors, and speech-language pathologists (Schow & Nerbonne, 2002). If the client has cognitive impairments in attention or memory due to dementia or AD or exhibits symptoms of depression with the dementia that further reduce cognitive abilities, then retaining any new information introduced during aural rehabilitation may be unlikely. Clients for whom a hearing aid or aids or assistive listening devices are prescribed may exhibit great difficulty using the devices correctly because of decreased cognitive abilities. Thus family member or caregiver involvement in the audiologic evaluation and aural rehabilitation process is highly recommended.

Family members and caregivers should be considered as integral team members who can provide additional medical information and client history to assist in the evaluation process. They may be able to provide more accurate descriptions of events and give examples of when hearing loss was first noted and any additional changes in hearing ability. Family members and caregivers can assist the audiologist by telling him or her what strategies seem to improve hearing in familiar environments. This information can greatly help the audiologist to evaluate hearing loss. In addition, family members or caregivers have frequent or daily

---

[*]From Brookshire, R. H. (2003). *Introduction to neurogenic communication disorders* (6th ed.). Reprinted with permission.

interactions with the individual with dementia or AD; thus they can provide valuable information about the client's communicative abilities.

After the audiologic evaluation, the client, family members, and caregivers are often provided with verbal information regarding the test results. Because of the cognitive changes of the client, information should be restated by using different modalities of communication. Education provided in different formats by the audiologist can also be beneficial to family members or caregivers. Educational and instructional information can be provided via handouts with pictures and written text. The information provided to the client with dementia or AD should be easy to understand and concise to assist with retention of any new information (Brookshire, 2003). Pictures on handouts should be clear and simple to aid in comprehension. Family members, caregivers, and the client can refer to the take-home materials if they have questions or require clarification.

In summary, the cognitive status of an individual with dementia should always be taken into account during an audiologic evaluation and aural rehabilitation. The ability to determine what is and is not working, what to do if something becomes problematic, when to ask for help, and whom to ask involves the use of cognitive functions. If any area in cognition is impaired, a presumably simple task can, in reality, be immensely difficult for an individual with dementia. Finally, family members or caregivers should be considered important team members who can supply information about functional hearing abilities and pertinent medical issues for the client with dementia.

ETHICS OF SERVICE PROVISION

The American Speech-Language-Hearing Association (ASHA) in 2003 provided audiologists and speech-language pathologists with a code of ethics by which they must abide. These principles and rules govern the services provided by these professionals. Guidelines are given for what constitutes professional competence, evaluation of the effectiveness of services, discussion of prognosis, and provision of services. As stated in the ASHA Code of Ethics (2003), individuals shall be provided services only when benefit can reasonably be expected. Thus if an individual with dementia or AD is provided for audiology or speech-language pathology services, it is imperative that the professional inform everyone involved with client care about what results can be realistically expected (Tanner, 2003).

The individual with dementia or AD may be able to participate actively in services by providing accurate verbal feedback during the mild or early stages of the disease. Services such as aural rehabilitation may be warranted in the early stages of dementia; however, as the disease progresses, professionals, family, or caregivers may instead choose to focus on quality of life. If a client with dementia either refuses to use an amplification device or cannot use one because of cognitive decline, then other means of communication must be investigated. Therefore the audiologist or speech-language pathologist working with the individual with dementia must use his or her knowledge and professional judgment when providing services. If professionals disregard the degenerative and progressive nature of the dementia and instead choose to provide unneeded or inadequate services that do not benefit the client, then he or she has breached the code of ethics (ASHA, 2003). If this occurs, a special board appointed by ASHA will review the case for the violation(s).

IDENTIFICATION AND EVALUATION OF DEMENTIA

Family members are often the first to recognize changes such as early symptoms of dementia in a loved one. For instance, a spouse may notice that his wife or her husband has difficulty recalling appointments, names of people, and familiar places. At times, the individual with dementia may feel anxious, frightened, or lost in his or her surroundings and notice that something is wrong. The individual may recognize subtle changes in his or her ability to recall new and recent information. These incidents may cause the individual or family to question whether the family member actually has dementia or whether another problem may be contributing to the change in cognition. When questions arise about dementia, a physician such as a neurologist, gerontologist, or related professional, such as a neuropsychologist, will use formal and informal examinations and standardized tests to determine whether the individual has dementia, the severity of the dementia, and the type of dementia. Of the evaluation tools available, the most frequently used screening tool to detect and determine severity of dementia is the Mini Mental

State Exam (MMSE) (Folstein, Folstein, & McHugh, 1975). The MMSE screens an individual for orientation to time and place, attention, receptive and expressive language, constructional abilities, and immediate and delayed memory. Scores on the MMSE are often used to determine the severity of cognitive deficits. For example, scores from 21 to 25 points indicate mild dementia, scores from 11 to 20 points indicate moderate dementia, and scores of 10 points or less indicate severe dementia. After the initial results of the MMSE, more in-depth neuropsychologic examinations that provide a more detailed picture of retained cognitive abilities can be administered.

In addition to the neuropsychologic tests, speech-language pathologists often use formal standardized tests to assess communication skills in individuals with dementia or AD. These tests include the Arizona Battery for Communication Disorders in Dementia (ABCD) (Bayles & Tomoeda, 1993) for individuals with mild to moderate AD and the Functional Linguistic Communication Inventory (FLCI) (Bayles & Tomoeda, 1994) for individuals with moderate to severe AD. The ABCD is designed to identify functional linguistic communication deficits associated with AD. The ABCD assists the clinician to evaluate orientation, immediate and delayed recall abilities, auditory comprehension, new learning, expressive language, reading comprehension, generative naming, semantic knowledge, and drawing. The clinician can give the test at different stages of dementia to determine what cognitive and communicative skills an individual retains and what skills have changed. The results can provide valuable information about what strategies to implement in the client's life to enhance his or her communication and daily activities. In addition, the results can assist family members to determine what can be done about safety issues for the client.

The FLCI is another commonly used test that assesses impairments in functional communication. This standardized test is used to evaluate clients in the later stages of dementia, particularly of the AD type. The areas examined in the FLCI include memory, expressive language, receptive language, writing, comprehension of signs, reading comprehension, pragmatics, and gestures. Results obtained from the FLCI can guide the clinician in counseling family or caregivers about the types of compensatory strategies needed to improve communication and quality of life.

Both the ABCD and the FLCI can provide valuable information about attention, memory, and auditory comprehension abilities. If, indeed, a client has problems with cognition and communication rather than an actual hearing loss, standardized tests and an auditory assessment can assist to identify the difference. Therefore working with other health care professionals as a team to determine whether a true hearing loss exists or whether the problem is actually related to a decrease in cognition and communication is essential in the care of an individual with dementia or AD.

In addition to the screening tools and formal evaluation tests used to detect changes in cognition and communication, the Global Deterioration Scale (GDS) (Reisberg, Ferris, de Leon, & Crook, 1982) is often used to categorize an individual's dementia or AD into the mild, moderate, or severe stages of disease progression. The GDS involves observations of a client with dementia; therefore scoring is based on the subjective judgment of the observer. Seven stages of cognitive decline are described with scores of 2 to 3 corresponding to the mild stages of the disease, 4 to 5 indicating moderate stages, and 6 to 7 associated with the severe stages of the disease. A score of 1 indicates that the client is functioning normally without any cognitive decline being observed. An individual with dementia in the mild stages often exhibits difficulties in working (short-term) and episodic (event) memory involved with the retention of new information (Hopper et al., 2001). For instance, an individual may forget his or her destination of travel or directions to reach the destination. This change in memory function can cause the individual with dementia to become afraid and fearful. Later in the mild stage, memory skills become progressively worse. Problems can occur with the ability to recall names of new people and remember new locations. In addition, attention and word retrieval skills may become impaired, but the individual should be able to continue interacting socially. Anxiety about changes in cognitive abilities may also be observed. Because of the cognitive and communicative changes involved, the individual may begin displaying some difficulty functioning in his or her work environments.

During the mild stages of dementia identified using the GDS, an audiologic referral and formal assessment for hearing ability would assist the client if any problems were noted. The individual with dementia or AD would be able to participate actively in the formal audiologic assessment during the mild stages. If amplification for hearing loss was recommended after the assessment, the use of a hearing aid or aids or listening device would assist the client by improving hearing function for comprehension of communication. This change would benefit the client in his or her familiar and unfamiliar surroundings for everyday activities. However, as the client's dementia or AD progresses, supervision may be needed to assist the client to recall where and how to store the device, how to use the hearing device properly (i.e., adjusting the volume and changing the batteries), and what to do if problems arise with the device.

During the moderate stages of dementia, the client may exhibit increased deficits in working and episodic memory (Hopper et al., 2001). For instance, events that occurred recently, such as going to a doctor's appointment or visiting a friend, may not be recalled. Reisberg et al. (1982) stated that problems could also be detected in attention, orientation, judgment, and problem solving. Familiar activities such as paying household bills may not be completed. During stage 5, the client will require supervision and outside assistance to maintain personal safety and to perform activities of daily living (Reisberg et al., 1982). Familiar information, such as the client's address, will not be recalled. Supervision will be required when the client uses any hearing amplification device during the moderate stages of dementia. Continued assistance will be required to use and care for the hearing device correctly. Any recommendations made by the audiologist or other professionals involved in aural rehabilitation will require the assistance of family or caregivers for follow-through.

Finally, in the severe stages of dementia, cognitive and communication skills continue to deteriorate, and the individual will require assistance for daily care (Reisberg et al., 1982). Individuals with dementia in the severe stages begin to forget the names of familiar family members and long-term personal information. Changes begin to emerge in personality, behavior, and emotion. For instance, the individual may act out violently toward family members or caregivers. Reisberg et al. (1982) reported that during stage 7, the client would lose all ability to communicate and require constant care for activities of daily living such as eating and toileting. The authors also stated that the physical ability to walk would be lost during this stage. Thus the use of an amplification device for hearing may not be ethically warranted during the later stages of disease unless the device improves quality of life. When the client is unable to comprehend information because of cognitive decline, amplifying the client's hearing will not change his or her comprehension abilities. Therefore during the severe stages of the disease, the focus should be on providing comfort to the client.

MANAGEMENT

As previously reviewed, when individuals age, high-frequency hearing loss is often encountered (National Institute on Aging, 2002). Thus audiologic evaluations should be completed regularly to determine whether any aural intervention or rehabilitation is necessary. In addition, if hearing assessments are completed regularly, the audiologist can monitor any changes in hearing ability. Therefore hearing assessment should also be done, even though an individual has the diagnosis of dementia or AD. Family members, along with physicians and health care professionals, must work as a team if they suspect that an individual with dementia or AD has a hearing loss (Schow & Nerbonne, 2002). At times it can be difficult to determine whether the hearing loss is affecting communication and comprehension of language or whether the actual reason stems from overall cognitive decline. Therefore if a hearing loss is identified in individuals with dementia or AD within the mild or early stages of the disease, then an active dialogue can occur between the audiologist and client.

As an individual progressively loses his or her cognitive abilities, less accurate information, decreased interaction, and participation are expected from the client. For instance, the client may experience difficulty in active participation in an audiologic evaluation because of changes in emotion, memory, and attention. If specific directions are provided to the client, he or she may forget the instructions and become easily distracted. Therefore several short evaluation sessions may be necessary to determine the hearing status of an individual with dementia or AD. Furthermore, family members and other health care professionals who have interacted often with the client may be able to provide information about the circumstances in which hearing appears to be most difficult for the client.

Because of possible difficulties in cognition, communication, emotion, and behavior of clients with dementia or AD, obtaining services from an audiologist with experience working with individuals with neurogenic disorders is highly recommended. The professional with this type of experience should provide the most effective and efficient services. In addition, he or she would be more capable of determining whether the client truly has a hearing loss or whether language comprehension is deteriorating because of cognitive decline. Thus an audiologist with a background in neurogenic disorders will be able to complete a thorough and accurate audiologic evaluation because of his or her experience working with challenging populations.

After the formal hearing evaluation, suggestions will be made about aural rehabilitation. Audiologists and other professionals can assist the client, family members, or caregivers with the implementation of the recommendations. Schow and Nerbonne (2002) reviewed the use of "CARE" for management in aural rehabilitation. CARE incorporates counseling, audibility and instrumental interventions, remediation for communication of activities, and environmental coordination and participation improvement (Schow & Nerbonne, 2002, p. 355). The audiologist is the first professional who will counsel an individual with dementia or AD and his or her family members or caregivers about hearing loss. Counseling should involve a thorough review of the audiologic test results and address the needs of the client. Furthermore, suggestions or recommendations about what can be done to improve hearing should be discussed. Questions or concerns posed by the client, family members, or caregivers can be discussed during the counseling session. In addition, counseling for individuals with dementia or AD should involve a review of the progression of the disease, effects of cognitive decline on language, and an explanation of how hearing loss can be affected by these changes. The counseling session should assist the client, family members, or caregivers to make decisions about how hearing loss can affect daily functioning and to determine which amplification device, if any, would promote the best hearing. Time spent counseling is important if the client, family members, or caregivers are still grieving over the diagnosis of dementia, continue to be in denial about the progressive nature of the disease, or exhibit stress over the changing responsibilities in family dynamics (Tanner, 2003). Thus it appears that a large quantity of information must be provided during counseling sessions, and it is better when a number of professionals work as a team to review the information about the diagnosis of dementia or AD and its effects on cognition and communication. This open interaction about dementia or AD will be beneficial to the client, family members, or caregivers when one obtains accurate information about any type of therapeutic service.

The second portion of CARE involves audibility and instrumental interventions (Schow & Nerbonne, 2002). If the audiologist recommends the use of a hearing aid or aids or other external amplification device early in the diagnosis of dementia or AD, family members, health care professionals, and the client must support the use of the device (Schow & Nerbonne, 2002). A hearing aid would provide the amplification needed by the individual with dementia or AD; however, the small size of the device can be extremely problematic. A hearing aid or aids may be easily lost or misplaced by the individual with dementia or his or her caregivers. Elderly adults may have difficulty manually manipulating the small device to adjust the volume or change batteries if assistance is unavailable. In addition to the size of the device being a barrier, if the amplification of sounds is perceived negatively when the device is used, then the individual with dementia may choose not to wear the device. This can occur if the sounds during conversation and within the environment seem too loud for the client to tolerate. Although these barriers exist for the use of amplification devices, a study by Allen et al. (2003) found that patients with dementia and hearing impairment benefited from the provision of hearing aids. In addition, both caregivers and patients noted improvements in hearing; however, no changes were found in cognitive function, activities of daily living, or caregiver burden.

External amplification devices such as hearing aids can assist individuals by increasing the intensity of sounds. Some disadvantages to purchasing a hearing aid include cost, lack of insurance coverage, and misunderstanding about the fact that the device will not work in all environments (National Institute on Aging, 2002). Other devices such as telephone amplification systems, assistive listening devices, and TV and radio listening systems are available to assist an individual with hearing loss. Similarly, the use of these systems depends on the daily activities and cognitive abilities of the individual with dementia or AD. As the disease progresses, amplification will not always be helpful to the client; rather it can become bothersome, or devices can become too difficult to use.

Finally, the remediation for communication activities and environmental coordination and participation improvement portions of CARE include practical suggestions of when and how to improve hearing ability (Schow & Nerbonne, 2002). For example, simple environmental changes can be incorporated into the client's life. By decreasing the noise level within the environment or decreasing the proximity between speaker and listener, positive changes in hearing abilities for communication can occur. Additional management suggestions include having the conversational partner(s) speak clearly, interacting face-to-face with conversational partners, providing concise information, simplifying communication as needed, providing repetition of information, and using multiple modalities for communication (National Institute on Aging, 2002). Multiple modalities used to enhance comprehension can include additional forms of communication such as the use of gestures, nonverbal communication, and writing (Brookshire, 2003). These simple suggestions can greatly improve communication with an individual with dementia or AD who has a hearing loss. These suggestions are also beneficial for other individuals who have neurogenic disorders and can be incorporated into the client's daily life to improve auditory comprehension. No matter what devices or strategies are involved in a client's aural rehabilitation, the focus of professional care should be on improving quality of life. As the disease progresses in an individual with dementia or AD, assisting the client to function to the best of his or her abilities is key.

SUMMARY

Dementia is a broad medical term encompassing different types of progressive degenerative diseases. Of the various types of dementia, Alzheimer's disease (AD) is the type identified most often. In dementia and AD, gradual changes occur in the areas of cognition, communication, physical abilities, behavior, and emotion. Because of the heterogeneity of individuals with dementia or AD, the length of time for progression through the stages of the disease and the severity of the disease can vary. Although medications are available to slow the rate of progression of the disease, it is important to remember that a cure is still unavailable.

Similar to the normal aging population, individuals with dementia or AD can also exhibit hearing loss. Although similar types of hearing loss may be evident in the individual with dementia or AD, the progressive loss of cognitive abilities can make the identification of an actual hearing loss more difficult, especially if a hearing evaluation is done in the moderate or middle stages of the disease. Thus a team approach involving the client, family members, caregivers, and health care professionals will ensure the best care possible. The audiologist will determine whether an actual hearing loss exists, and information obtained by family members, caregivers, and other professionals can assist to determine whether language comprehension problems stem from cognitive decline or from an actual hearing loss. After the audiologic evaluation, aural rehabilitation will require the assistance of all team members to carry out the recommendations made by the audiologist. The use of hearing devices and listening strategies will have to be monitored and modified as cognitive and communicative changes occur in the client. Finally, professionals working with individuals with dementia or AD should always keep in mind that the most important goal is to improve the client's quality of life.

ACKNOWLEDGMENTS

The author would like to thank Joanne Kawahigashi Oshiro, M.S., CCC-SLP, for her editing remarks and encouragement to complete this chapter. In addition, the author would like to thank Kenneth Pugh, Ph.D., CCC-Aud, for his motivating words and advice during the writing process.

REFERENCES

Allen, N. H., Burns, A., Newton, V., Hickson, F., Ramsden, R., Rogers, J., et al. (2003). The effects of improving hearing in dementia. *Age and Ageing, 32,* 189–193.

Alzheimer's Association. (2003). *About Alzheimer's.* Retrieved August 30, 2004, from http://www.alz.org/AboutAD/overview.htm.

American Psychiatric Association. (1994). *Diagnostic and statistical manual of mental disorders* (4th ed.). Washington, DC: Author.

American Speech-Language-Hearing Association. (2003). ASHA code of ethics (revised). *ASHA Supplement, 23,* 13–15.

Bayles, K. A., & Tomoeda, C. K. (1993). *The Arizona Battery of Communication Disorders of Dementia.* Austin, TX: PRO-ED.

Bayles, K. A., & Tomoeda, C. K. (1994). *Functional Linguistic Communication Inventory.* Austin, TX: PRO-ED.

Brookshire, R. H. (2003). *Introduction to neurogenic communication disorders* (6th ed.). St. Louis: Mosby.

Dementia. (2003, March 26). Retrieved July 30, 2003, from http://www.neurologychannel. com/dementia/.

Folstein, M. F., Folstein, S. E., & McHugh, P. R. (1975). "Mini-mental state." A practical method for grading the cognitive state of patients for the clinician. *Journal of Psychiatric Research, 12,* 189–198.

Hopper, T., Bayles, K. A., & Kim, E. (2001). Retained neuropsychological abilities of individuals with Alzheimer's disease. *Seminar in Speech and Language, 22,* 261–273.

National Institute on Aging Information Center (2002, September).

Hearing loss (National Institute on Aging Health Information AgePage). Retrieved August 1, 2003, from http://www.nia.nih.gov/health/agepages/hearing.htm.

Reisberg, B., Ferris, S. H., de Leon, M. J., & Crook, T. (1982). The global deterioration scale for assessment of primary degenerative dementia. *American Journal of Psychiatry, 139,* 1136–1139.

Schow, R. L, & Nerbonne, M. A. (2002). *Introduction to audiologic rehabilitation* (4th ed.). Boston: Allyn & Bacon.

Tanner, D. C. (2003). *The psychology of neurogenic communication disorders, a primer for health care professionals.* Boston: Allyn & Bacon.

Weinstein, B. E. (2000). *Geriatric audiology.* New York: Thieme Medical Publishers.

CHAPTER 6

Otitis Media: Diagnosis and Management

Teralandur K. Parthasarathy, Ph.D.
Department of Special Education and Communication Disorders
Southern Illinois University Edwardsville
Edwardsville, IL

Gita J. Malur, M.D.
Pediatic Healthcare Unlimited
Alton, IL

Otitis media (OM) is a major cause of auditory dysfunction in preschool and early grade school children. At especially high risk are children with Turner's, Apert's, or Down's syndromes or cleft palate/lip or any maxillofacial malformation and some groups of mentally retarded children. Between 26 and 43% of the population with mental retardation and developmental disabilities caused by Down's syndrome have a higher incidence of OM than the remaining mentally retarded and developmentally disabled population. Early detection and aggressive multidisciplinary assessment and management are critical to minimize the long-term adverse effects of hearing impairment on aspects of central auditory function or processing, linguistic–cognitive function, and educational attainment.

Few medical conditions are as common or as frustrating as OM. Because it can result in impaired hearing during the critical years of speech and language development, the increasing incidence of OM is of major concern to parents, pediatricians, family physicians, and otolaryngologists. Nothing about it is easy: The diagnosis is challenging, the range of management options perplexing, and the array of medications and regimens daunting.

OM refers to an inflammation of the middle ear cavity without reference to etiology or pathogenesis. It is one of the most common conditions diagnosed by pediatricians in the United States, and its incidence in children is growing (Schappert, 1992). Direct and indirect costs associated with OM have been estimated to be in the billions of dollars per year (Stool, Berg, & Berman, 1994; Stool & Field, 1989). It occurs more often in children than in adults, and its incidence seems to decrease with age (Teele, Klein, & Rosner, 1989; Wright, McConnel, & Thompson).

This chapter focuses on the definition, pathogenesis, and diagnostic and management options for OM, a common but complex condition of infants and children in the United States.

DEFINITION

Otitis media is a general term that encompasses an array of disease processes (Paparella, Bluestone, & Arnold, 1985). The term *acute otitis media* (*AOM*) refers to an acute inflammation of the middle ear with a rapid onset of one or more symptoms such as ear pain, ear pulling, otorrhea, fever, irritability, vomiting, and diarrhea. In patients with AOM, the tympanic membrane (TM) will eventually bulge with limited or no mobility to pneumatic otoscopy, which is indicative of *middle ear effusion (MEE)*. Redness of the TM without MEE is called *myringitis* and is often mistaken for AOM (Stool et al., 1994).

MEE is a fluid in the middle ear space. An effusion may be (1) *mucoid* (a thick, viscous, mucuslike liquid), (2) *serous* (a thin, watery liquid), (3) *purulent* (a puslike liquid), or (4) a combination of all three.

MEE can be the result of either AOM or OM with effusion (Bluestone, 1994; Bluestone & Klein, 1995). Approximately 70% of all children in this country will have an occurrence by age 3 years, making it the most common diagnosis in the pediatrician's office.

Otitis media with effusion (OME) is an inflammation of the middle ear in which the acute infection has resolved, but fluid in the middle ear space persists, sometimes for prolonged periods (Stool et al., 1994). Diagnosis of OME requires assessment of middle ear function by means of pneumatic otoscopy or tympanometry (Stool et al., 1994).

Many synonymous terms are used to describe asymptomatic effusion in the middle ear, such as serous OM, secretory OM, and non-suppurative OM, but the commonly accepted term is OME (Stool et al., 1994).

The term *persistent middle ear effusion* refers to asymptomatic effusion that persists for weeks to months or months after the onset of AOM. The term *chronic otitis media with effusion (COME)* is used when MEE persists for 4 months or longer after onset of AOM (Stool et al., 1994). Risk factors for COME are shown in Table 6.1.

PATHOGENESIS

The pathogenesis of OM is multifactorial (see Table 6.1), including predisposing factors, host-related factors, and non–host-related factors (Casselbrant, Mandel, & Fall, 1999; Teele et al., 1989). An immature immune system and a functionally immature eustachian tube are the two most common factors related to the increased incidence of OM in infants and young children.

In most children and infants, eustachian tube dysfunction is most commonly caused by viral infection of the upper respiratory tract. The most important function of the eustachian tube is ventilation of the middle ear cavity. In the presence of eustachian tube dysfunction, the trapped air in the middle cavity is absorbed, creating negative pressure, retraction of the TM, fluid accumulation in the middle ear, and, eventually, bacterial invasion and proliferation (Daly, Hunter, & Giebink, 1999).

It has been well established that a high incidence (45–54%) of persistent conductive hearing impairment compared with that in the

Table 6.1

Risk Factors for Chronic Otitis Media with Effusion

Predisposing Factors	Host-Related Factors	Non–Host-Related Factors
Maxillofacial abnormalities	Male gender	Group day-care attendance
Eustachian tube dysfunction	Race (Canadian, Eskimo, or Native American)	Passive smoke exposure
Immunologic deficiencies	Sibling history or recurrent AOM	Bottle feeding
	Early onset (before age 2 years) of first occurrence	Use of pacifier
		Socioeconomic conditions Genetics

From Parthasarathy, T. K., Bhat, V., & Malur, G. J. (2003). Otitis media: A primer on diagnosis and management. *The Hearing Journal, 56*(6): 42–48. (Reprinted with permission from *The Hearing Journal* and Lippincott Williams & Wilkins.)

general population is seen in children with Turner's, Apert's, or Down's syndrome, cleft palate/lip, any maxillofacial malformation, or some groups of mentally retarded children because of clear anatomic differences in the head and neck region.

Whereas viruses typically are present before AOM and commonly exist as copathogens, they are the sole pathogen in only in a small percentage (6–7%) of children with AOM. *Streptococcus pneumoniae* is the most common pathogen, followed by *Haemophilus influenzae* and *Moraxella catarrhalis* (Bluestone, Stephenson, & Martin, 1992). Thus the isolation of a specific pathogen may assist in the use of appropriate antibiotics to treat the AOM. Spontaneous resolution of AOM and OME occurs in 80–90% of all patients within 3 months of onset (Stool et al., 1994).

DIAGNOSIS AND IMPLICATIONS

Accurate diagnosis of AOM is critical for appropriate treatment and follow-up. However, accurate diagnosis is often difficult in infants and young children. Symptoms of AOM are less apparent or absent or, most often, overlap with those of upper respiratory tract infections. Additional challenges include lack of patient cooperation, excessive cerumen in the external auditory canal, and stenosis of the external auditory canal. Inexperience in the removal of cerumen and in pneumatic otoscopy also contributes to inaccurate diagnoses (Hoberman, Paradise, & Wald, 1997).

Pneumatic otoscopy is a simple and inexpensive procedure to evaluate the status of the TM for *contour* (normal, retracted, full, or bulging), *color* (yellow, gray, pink, amber, red, white, or blue), *translucency,* and *mobility.* In questionable instances, results can be verified by performing tympanometry, which has higher specificity than pneumatic otoscopy in detecting OME (Daly et al., 1999).

Tympanocentesis, which involves puncturing the TM and aspirating middle ear fluid to permit the identification of pathogens, has greater clinical significance in selection of the optimal antimicrobial therapy (Hoberman et al., 1997). Diagnostic tympanocentesis is strongly indicated when symptoms of AOM fail to resolve after the first and second courses of antibiotic treatment.

For many years, numerous antibiotics were available for treatment of middle ear infections, and all appeared to be relatively effective. However, in the past decade, the emergence of resistance to antibiotics among the common otitic pathogens and increased incidence of recurrent AOM in infants in day care have complicated the selection of antimicrobial therapy (Hoberman et al., 1997).

In 1994, a task force including the Agency for Health Care Policy and Research (AHCPR) (Stool et al., 1994), in collaboration with the American Academy of Pediatrics, the American Academy of Physicians, and the American Academy of Otolaryngology, prepared specific guidelines for the management of OME in children between age 1 and 3 years (Stool et al., 1994). The task force panel concluded that when OME is suspected, pneumatic otoscopy or tympanometry should be performed to confirm the presence of effusion and to determine TM mobility. After confirmation of OME, parental counseling and education about the risk factors listed in Table 6.1 should be provided, and the child should be reexamined in 6 weeks. The AHCPR algorithm (Figs. 6.1 and 6.2) is recommended for managing OME in an otherwise healthy child between age 1 and 3 years (Stool et al., 1994).

The AHCPR guideline provides an excellent, comprehensive review of the scientific literature on OME. It has, however, been criticized for being narrow in scope, favoring medical as opposed to surgical management of OME. Thus children between age 1 and 3 years who are at risk for experiencing recurrent AOM (see Table 6.1) may require more aggressive medical or surgical management (Bluestone & Klein, 1995).

Most cases of OME are associated with a transient conductive hearing loss averaging about 25 dB hearing level (HL) (Rosenfield et al., 1994). The amount and viscosity of fluid in the middle ear determine the degree and configuration of hearing loss (Gravel & Ellis, 1995; Gravel & Wallace, 2000). In some children, there is an increased risk of a permanent high-frequency sensorineural hearing loss (Hunter et al., 1996). The mild, recurrent hearing loss, rather than OME, seems to have an adverse effect on aspects of central auditory function or processing, linguistic-cognitive function, and educational attainment (Gravel & Wallace, 1992, 1995).

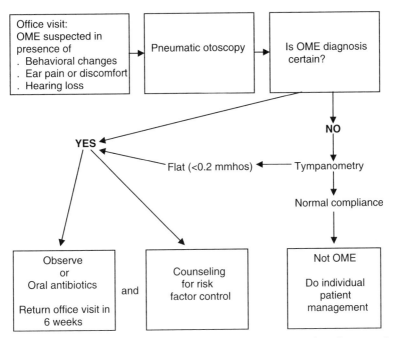

Figure 6.1 Agency for Health Care Policy and Research algorithm for managing otitis media with effusion (OME). (From Parthasarathy, T. K., Bhat, V., & Malur, G. J. [2003]. Otitis media: A primer on diagnosis and management. *The Hearing Journal, 56*[6]: 42–48. Reprinted with permission from *The Hearing Journal* and Lippincott Williams & Wilkins.)

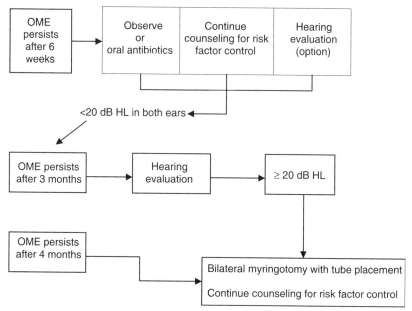

Figure 6.2   Agency for Health Care Policy and Research algorithm for managing persistent otitis media with effusion (OME). (From Parthasarathy, T. K., Bhat, V., & Malur, G. J. [2003]. Otitis media: A primer on diagnosis and management. *The Hearing Journal, 56*[6]: 42–48. Reprinted with permission from *The Hearing Journal* and Lippincott Williams & Wilkins.)

Table 6.2

Medical Complications of Untreated Chronic Otitis Media with Effusion

Intracranial	Extracranial
Abscess	Tympanic membrane perforation
Extradural	Cholesteatoma
Subdural	Mastoiditis
Brain	Tympanosclerosis
Meningitis	Ossicular discontinuity
Lateral sinus thrombosis	Facial paralysis
Otic hydrocephalus	Labyrinthitis
	Hearing impairment
	Conductive (most common)
	Mixed
	Sensorineural

From Parthasarathy, T. K., Bhat, V., & Malur, G. J. (2003). Otitis media: A primer on diagnosis and management. *The Hearing Journal, 56*(6): 42–48. (Reprinted with permission from *The Hearing Journal* and Lippincott Williams & Wilkins.)

MANAGEMENT

Medical treatment is the first line of defense for children with OME. Currently, with use of antibiotics, some of the potential complications of untreated OME (Table 6.2) are uncommon.

Most children with AOM are treated with an antimicrobial agent (Table 6.3). All such medications have approximately equivalent clinical efficacy, although there are significant differences in their cost, side effects, and palatability.

Amoxicillin at 40–60 mg/kg/day remains the first standard line of treatment in most children (Doern, Brueggemann, & Pierce, 1997). This drug is relatively safe and inexpensive, is well tolerated, and is effective against the gram-positive bacteria *S. pneumoniae*. However, two gram-negative pathogens—β-lactamase producing *H. influenzae* and *M. catarrhalis*—are resistant to amoxicillin treatment (Doern et al., 1997).

In children with persistent AOM or at high risk for COME based on host and nonhost factors (see Table 6.1), it may be preferable to start treatment with a drug or combination of drugs that is effective against the three most common pathogens: *S. pneumoniae, H. influenzae, and M. catarrhalis* (Barnett, Teele, & Klein, 1997). Such agents include second- and third-generation cephalosporins (see Table 6.3), which are effective against gram-negative bacteria, including *H. influenzae* and *M. catarrhalis*. They have been widely used for the treatment of upper and lower respiratory tract infections, sinusitis, and AOM (Barnett et al., 1997).

In some children, higher-than-standard dosages of amoxicillin (e.g., 80–100 mg/kg/day) are recommended. This approach is based on pharmacokinetic studies that suggest higher dosages of amoxicillin are more active against moderately and highly resistant *S. pneumoniae* (Block, 1997; McCraken, 1995). Linsk, Gilsdorf, & Lesperance (1999) developed a management approach for patients with a high risk of having amoxicillin-resistant *S. pneumoniae* (Fig. 6.3).

Currently, there is no consensus as to what constitutes amoxicillin treatment failure. Linsk et al. (1999) defined amoxicillin treatment failure as the "persistence or rapid recurrence of OM symptoms, such as otalgia, irritability, sleeplessness, anorexia or fever, together with physical

Table 6.3

Available Antimicrobial Agents for the Treatment of Acute Otitis Media

First-line agents
Aminopenicillin
  Amoxicillin

Second-line agents
Aminopenicillin plus β-lactamase inhibitor
  Amoxicillin–clavulanate

Cephalosporins (second-generation)
  Cefaclor
  Cefprozil
  Cefuroxime
  Cefixime
  Loracarbef

Cephalosporins (third-generation)
  Cefpodoxime
  Cefdinir
  Ceftibuten
  Ceftriaxone (intramuscular)

Macrolides
  Azithromycin
  Erythromycin–sulfisoxazole
  Clarithromycin

Trimethoprim-sulfamethoxazole (TMP-SMX)
Fluroquinolones
  Ofloxacin (otic drops for AOM in patients with tympanostomy tubes)

From Parthasarathy, T. K., Bhat, V., & Malur, G. J. (2003). Otitis media: A primer on diagnosis and management. *The Hearing Journal, 56*(6): 42–48. (Reprinted with permission from *The Hearing Journal* and Lippincott Williams & Wilkins.)

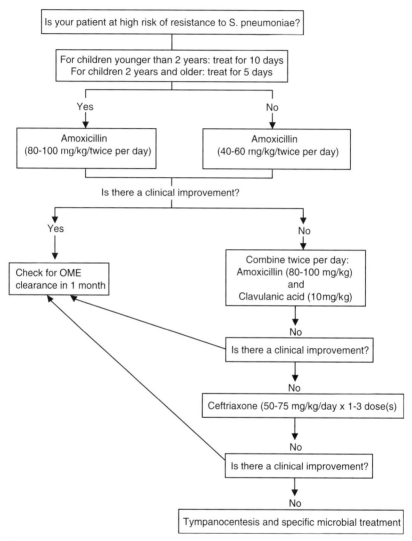

Figure 6.3   Acute otitis media (AOM) treatment approach. *OME*, otitis media with effusion (From Parthasarathy, T. K., Bhat, V., & Malur, G. J. [2003]. Otitis media: A primer on diagnosis and management. *The Hearing Journal, 56*[6]: 42–48. Reprinted with permission from *The Hearing Journal* and Lippincott Williams & Wilkins.)

findings of an inflamed tympanic membrane and middle ear effusion, in a patient who has received a dose of 40 to 60 mg/kg/day of amoxicillin for at least 72 hours" (p. 71).

Drug Treatment No Longer Automatic

Propelled by evidence-based medicine, the treatment paradigm for OME is changing, and medications are no longer automatically prescribed. Now, selective rather than routine use of antibiotics is preferred, largely because spontaneous resolution of AOM and OME is so common.

The increasing resistance of *S. pneumoniae, H. influenzae,* and *M. catarrhalis* to antibiotics has made treatment of OM more difficult. This factor, coupled with the growing recognition of the role of viruses, has stimulated efforts to *prevent* rather than to *treat* OME. Accordingly, a new generation of protein conjugate *S. pneumoniae* bacterial vaccines that shows promise in the prevention of OM was recently approved by the U.S. Food and Drug Administration for use in children (Black, Shinefield, & Fireman, 2000).

Several investigators have evaluated the efficacy of shorter courses of antibiotic treatment in AOM. At present, the only oral drug approved for use in a 5-day regimen is azithromycin. Double-blind studies have shown that the outcome of a 5-day intake of azithromycin is equivalent to 10 days of amoxicillin-clavulanate (Pichichero & Cohen, 1997).

Surgical Treatment

When pharmaceutical treatment options have been exhausted, surgery must be considered. In the past decade, as an increasing percentage of middle ear organisms have become resistant to antibiotics, surgical treatment of OME has taken on new importance. Referral to an otolaryngologist should be considered after 3 months of bilateral OME, particularly when there is no evidence of improvement and when hearing loss is suspected (see Fig. 6.2) (Stool et al., 1994). The many factors that favor surgical treatment of OME (Stool et al., 1994) are shown in Table 6.4.

Table 6.4

Factors Favoring Surgical Treatment of Chronic Otitis Media with Effusion

Bilateral disease
Bilateral hearing loss (20 dB hearing threshold level [HTL] or greater)
Significant speech–language deficits
Behavioral problems
Tympanic membrane retraction
Ear pain or pulling
Recurrent AOM
Antibiotic allergies
Frequent smoke exposure
Group day care
Persistent AOM (3 months or longer)

From Parthasarathy, T. K., Bhat, V., & Malur, G. J. (2003). Otitis media: A primer on diagnosis and management. *The Hearing Journal, 56*(6): 42–48. (Reprinted with permission from *The Hearing Journal* and Lippincott Williams & Wilkins.)

More than 500,000 children a year in the United States undergo tympanostomy tube placement for chronic OME. The AHCPR guidelines (see Fig. 6.2) recommend that a child who has persistent OME for 4–6 months and who presents with a bilateral hearing loss (20 dB hearing threshold level [HTL] or greater) should have a bilateral myringotomy with tube placement. The AHCPR did not recommend adenoidectomy as a treatment for OME in young children between age 1 and 3 years (Stool et al., 1994). In addition, there is little evidence that either myringotomy alone or tonsillectomy has any significant place in the management of OME. The use of steroids, antihistamines, and decongestant medications is also not recommended in the management of OME (Stool et al., 1994).

AUDIOLOGIC MANAGEMENT CONSIDERATIONS

The educational implications of mild, fluctuating, conductive hearing impairment are significant and must be considered in the management of OME. The audiologic management considerations for OME should include (1) information about auditory-based communication strategies, (2) information about auditory behaviors that might signal OM infection, and (3) information about classroom accommodations, such as preferential seating, peer assistance, decreasing noise floor in the classroom, and sound field amplification systems.

Management of OME, like assessment, should be multidisciplinary. Audiologists, speech-language pathologists, pediatricians, otolaryngologists, teachers, and parents should be involved in the child's overall care.

The American Academy of Audiology (AAA) in 1992 issued a position statement recommending a three-step guideline (Table 6.5) for children with persistent learning and communication deficits related to untreated or undetected OM. The AAA developed additional guidelines in 1997, and the American Speech-Language-Hearing Association in 1993 developed a comprehensive management program for school-age children with undetected or untreated OM.

A few children are already at risk for learning and language problems such as those from special populations with Turner's, Apert's, or Down's syndrome, cleft palate/lip, any maxillofacial malformation, and some groups of mentally retarded children (Roberts & Hunter, 2002).

Table 6.5

American Academy of Audiology Audiologic Guidelines for Managing Otitis Media with Effusion

Identification Process	Assessment Process	Management Process
Screening for hearing, middle ear function, and speech and language development	Diagnostic audiologic assessment (pure tone, speech audiometry, acoustic, immittance, and formal language assessment)	Audiometric monitoring at least once during winter months
	Central auditory processing evaluation when indicated	Counseling to parents, caregivers, and teachers on implications of hearing impairment on communication

From Parthasarathy, T. K., Bhat, V., & Malur, G. J. (2003). Otitis media: A primer on diagnosis and management. *The Hearing Journal, 56*(6): 42–48. (Reprinted with permission from *The Hearing Journal* and Lippincott Williams & Wilkins.)

Early detection and aggressive multidisciplinary assessment and management are critical to minimize the long-term adverse effects of hearing impairment on aspects of central auditory function or processing, linguistic-cognitive function, and educational attainment.

Screening of children with OME for academic or developmental deficits is critical. The Early Language Milestone (ELM) scale can be useful to identify deficits in young children between age 1 and 3 years (Coplan, 1987). For identifying school-age children who are at risk in the classroom, the Screening Instrument for Targeting Educational Risk (SIFTER) (Anderson, 1989) can be very beneficial.

SUMMARY

The incidence of AOM in children has increased during the past decade. The most common organisms causing AOM in children in the United States are *S. pneumoniae, H. influenzae,* and *M. catarrhalis.* Resistance of these pathogens to antibiotics has also increased during the past decade. Because of this, the treatment paradigm for AOM is changing. Drug treatment is no longer automatic. Evidence-based medicine is helping to propel this paradigm shift in treating AOM so that selective rather than routine use of antibiotics is preferred.

Many factors contribute to an increased risk of development of AOM in children. By clearly understanding the role these factors play and the variations in resistance patterns of bacterial pathogens in each geographic community, an optimal treatment plan can be developed for patients with AOM.

Environmental modifications, immunizations, and pharmaceutical and surgical options should be considered. Pediatricians and family care physicians can play an active role by educating parents about risk factors for AOM and how to minimize their effects. Given the potential long-term impact that fluctuating OME-caused hearing impairment can have on central auditory function, linguistic-cognitive function, and educational attainment, audiologists must be vigilant and proactive to provide professional services for the early detection and nonmedical management of OM.

Management of OME, like assessment, should be multidisciplinary. Audiologists, speech-language pathologists, pediatricians, otolaryngologists, teachers, and parents should be involved in the child's overall care. Effective communication and partnership among audiologists, speech-language pathologists, day-care providers, parents, and primary care providers are critical in the overall management of OM.

REFERENCES

American Academy of Audiology. (1992). Position statement on guidelines for the diagnosis and treatment of otitis media in children. *Audiology Today, 4,* 23–24.

American Academy of Audiology. (1997). Identification of hearing loss and middle-ear dysfunction in preschool and school-aged children. *Audiology Today, 9,* 18–23.

American Speech-Language-Hearing Association (ASHA). (1993). Guidelines for audiology services in the schools. *ASHA Supplement, 35*(3), 24–32.

Anderson, K. L. (1989). *Screening instrument for targeting educational risk.* Danville, IL: Interstate.

Barnett, E. D., Teele, D. W., & Klein, J. O. (1997). Comparison of ceftriaxone and trimethoprim-sulfamethoxazole for acute otitis media. *Pediatrics, 99,* 23–28.

Black, S., Shinefield, H., & Fireman, B. (2000). Efficacy, safety and immmunogenicity of heptavalent pneumococcal conjugate vaccine in children. *The Pediatric Infectious Disease Journal, 19,* 187–195.

Block, S. L. (1997). Causative pathogens, antibiotic resistance and therapeutic considerations in acute otitis media. *The Pediatric Infectious Disease Journal, 16,* 449–456.

Bluestone, C. D. (1994). Surgical management of otitis media: Current indications and role related to increasing bacterial resistance. *The Pediatric Infectious Disease Journal, 13,* 1058–1063.

Bluestone, C. D., & Klein, J. O. (1995). *Otitis media in infants and children* (pp. 34–57). Philadelphia: Saunders.

Bluestone, C. D., Stephenson, J. S., & Martin, L. M. (1992). Ten year review of otitis media pathogens. *The Pediatric Infectious Disease Journal, 11,* 7–11.

Casselbrant, M. L., Mandel, E. M., & Fall, P. A. (1999). The heritability of otitis media: A twin and triplet study. *JAMA: The Journal of the American Medical Association, 282,* 2125–2130.

Coplan, J. (1987). *The Early Language Milestone Scale (ELM).* Austin, TX: PRO-ED.

Daly, K. A., Hunter, L. L., & Giebink, G. S. (1999). Chronic otitis media. *Pediatrics in Review, 20,* 85–93.

Doern, G. V., Brueggemann, A. B., & Pierce, G. (1997). Antibiotic resistance among clinical isolates of *Haemophilus influenzae* in the United States in 1994 and 1995 and detection of β-lactamase positive strains resistant to amoxicillin-clavulanate: Results of a national multicenter surveillance study. *Antimicrobial Agents and Chemotherapy, 41,* 292–297.

Gravel, J. S., & Ellis, M. A. (1995). Examining the auditory consequences of otitis media: The audiogram beyond. *Seminars in Hearing, 16*, 44–59.

Gravel, J. S., & Wallace, I. F. (1992). Listening and language at 4 years of age: Effects of early otitis media. *Journal of Speech and Hearing Research, 35*, 588–595.

Gravel, J. S., & Wallace, I. F. (1995). Early otitis media, auditory abilities, and educational risk. *American Journal of Speech-Language Pathology, 4*, 89–94.

Gravel, J. S., & Wallace, I. F. (2000). Effects of otitis media with effusion on hearing in the first 3 years of life. *Journal of Speech and Hearing Research, 43*, 631–644.

Hoberman, A., Paradise, J. L., & Wald, E. R. (1997). Tympanocentesis technique revisited. *The Pediatric Infectious Disease Journal, 16*(Suppl. 2), 25–26.

Hunter, L. L., Margolis, R. H., Ryyken, J. R., Le, C. T., Dayly, A., & Giebink, G. S. (1996). High frequency hearing loss associated with otitis media. *Ear and Hearing, 17*, 1–11.

Linsk, R., Gilsdorf, J., & Lesperance, M. (1999). When amoxicillin fails. *Contemporary Pediatrics, 16*, 67–88.

McCracken, G. H. (1995). Emergence of resistant *Streptococcus pneumoniae*: A problem in pediatrics. *The Pediatric Infectious Disease Journal, 14*, 424–428.

Paparella, M. M., Bluestone, C. D., & Arnold, W. (1985). Definition and classification. *Annals of Otology, Rhinology, and Laryngolology, 94*, 8–9.

Pichichero, M. E., & Cohen, R. (1997). Shortened course of antibiotic therapy for acute otitis media, sinusitis and tonsillopharyngitis. *The Pediatric Infectious Disease Journal, 16*, 680–695.

Roberts, J., & Hunter, L. (2002). Otitis media and children's language and learning. *ASHA Leader, 7*, 18–19.

Rosenfield, R. M., Vertrees, J. E., Carr, J., Cippole, R. J., Uden, D. L., Giebink, G. S., et al. (1994). Clinical efficacy of antimicrobial drugs for acute otitis media: Metaanalysis of 5400 children from thirty-three randomized trials. *Journal of Pediatrics, 124*, 355–367.

Schappert, S. M. (1992). Office visits for otitis media: United States, 1975–90. *National Center for Health Statistics, 214*, 1–18.

Stool, S. E., Berg, A. O. & Berman, S. (1994, July). *Otitis media with effusion in young children.* Clinical Practice Guideline No. 12 (AHCPR Publication No. 94-0622). Rockville, MD: U.S. Department of Health and Human Services.

Stool, S. E., & Field, M. J. (1989) The impact of otitis media. *The Pediatric Infectious Disease Journal, 8*, 11–14.

Teele, D. W., Klein, J. O., Rosner, B. A. (1989). Epidemiology of otitis media during the first seven years of life in children in greater Boston: a prospective, cohort study. *Journal of Infectious Disease, 160*, 83–94.

Wright, P. F., McConnel, K. B., & Thompson, J. M. (1985). A longitudinal study of the detection of otitis media in the first two years of life. *International Journal of Pediatric Otolaryngology, 10*, 245–252.

CHAPTER 7

Cerumen Management

John M.A. Oyiborhoro, Ed.D., F.A.A.A., CCC-A
Boro Audiology Clinic
Brooklyn, NY
and
National Institute for People with Disabilities
New York, NY

It is well documented that impacted cerumen is a common occurrence among consumers, especially those who are mentally retarded (Brister, Fullwood, Ripp, & Blodgett, 1986; Crandell & Roeser, 1993; Fulton & Griffin, 1967). In addition to the deleterious effects that impacted cerumen has on the consumer, the clinician has other practical concerns. A clear ear canal is important to perform several audiologic procedures. For instance, procedures such as the use of probe tips in immittance measures, use of insert earphones, taking of ear impressions for custom hearing aids or earmolds, obtaining of otoacoustic emissions (OAEs) and real ear measurements, and electronystagmography all require clear ear canals to be successfully and effectively completed. Excessive cerumen accumulation in the ear canal can be considered a fairly serious health issue among people with disabilities that needs to be attended to in rehabilitation.

Except for elderly persons, the incidence of impacted cerumen among consumers is much higher than that in the general population; it ranges between 22 and 36% (Brister et al., 1986; Crandell & Roeser, 1993; Fulton & Griffin, 1967; Nudo, 1965; Oyiborhoro, 1993).

WHAT IS CERUMEN?

Cerumen (earwax) is a viscous, sticky, and oily substance that covers the surface linings of the external auditory canal. Cerumen is produced from secretions of the sebaceous and ceruminous glands located in the cartilaginous portion of the external auditory canal. These secretions are mixed with dead epithelial cells and foreign bodies, such as dust, and form cerumen. Cerumen serves several useful protective functions: (1) It helps repel water and cleans and lubricates the external ear canal; (2) it helps to trap foreign bodies such as dust, dirt, and insects; and (3) it helps to protect the ear against possible bacterial invasion and fungal growth (Stone & Fulghum, 1984).

However, despite its protective functions, cerumen becomes a health issue among people with disabilities, particularly mentally retarded consumers, when its accumulation in the ear canal becomes excessive. Cerumen may become hard and dry due to atrophy of the ceruminous glands (Kirkwood, 1993). Cerumen impaction results when its natural state is altered and the material becomes hard, thereby slowing down or rendering its natural self-removal and cleaning mechanism during jaw movements—chewing, talking, or laughing—ineffective. Failure to efficiently remove excessive cerumen from the ear canal adds to further accumulation and build-up of the substance. Increased sebaceous and ceruminous glandular activities result in increased production of cerumen. Also, external ear canal abnormalities, such as those seen in Down's syndrome with its high incidence of stenotic (narrow) ear canals (Northern & Downs, 1984) or collapsible ear canals interfere with the normal self-cleansing of the external auditory canal. This causes excessive cerumen build-up and impaction in the ear canal.

IMPACT OF EXCESSIVE CERUMEN

One major consequence of excessive or impacted cerumen in the ear canal is that it is a common cause of conductive hearing impairment, especially among consumers with mental retardation (Bricco, 1985; Crandell & Roeser, 1993; Ruby, 1986). Excessive cerumen blocks or reduces the amount of sound that is transmitted to the inner ear through the external ear canal. The degree of the resulting conductive hearing loss depends on the amount of accumulated cerumen and blockage. Crandell and Roeser (1993) reported that 80% of ear canal occlusion may cause a mild degree of conductive hearing loss, whereas a completely occluded ear canal can cause a 40–45 dB conductive hearing impairment. Symptoms and other problems that are associated with impacted cerumen include, but are not limited to, tinnitus, dizziness, or vertigo; pain; itching; and otitis externa (inflammation of the external auditory canal) (Adams, Boies, & Papparella, 1978; Kirkwood, 1993).

As indicated earlier, the occurrence of impacted cerumen among consumers with mental retardation is considerably higher than that in the non–mentally retarded population (Crandell & Roeser, 1993; Nudo, 1965). For instance, Crandell and Roeser (1993) found an incidence of excessive and impacted cerumen of 28% in the mentally retarded population compared with an incidence of 2–6% in subjects from the general adult population. They concluded that the ears of individuals with mental retardation have more propensity to develop excessive cerumen and, thus, exhibit the attendant consequences of varying degrees of conductive hearing loss, including its impact on cognitive, social, and linguistic development. It is quite possible that greater amounts of cerumen are produced in mentally retarded consumers with other disabilities such as cerebral palsy than in non–mentally retarded consumers, but a lack of periodic audiologic services, which offer an opportunity for early identification of excessive wax build-up and necessary follow-up for cerumen management, to these consumers can also be a factor (Oyiborhoro, 1993). It is difficult for consumers with significant cognitive deficits or severe physical disabilities to maintain good aural hygiene without assistance. Because of the high incidence of excessive and impacted cerumen among consumers and the consequent audiologic and otologic sequelae, cerumen management should be considered an important health service issue.

In addition to causing conductive hearing loss and having an indirect impact on the cognitive, social, and linguistic development of consumers, excessive cerumen accumulation in the ear canal can also cause consumers to experience tinnitus, dizziness, itching, pain, and discomfort. Otitis externa can result from the presence of excessive cerumen in the ear canal.

Earlier studies in which high incidences of excessive cerumen among mentally retarded consumers were investigated involved subjects who were selected from institutionalized populations (Fulton & Griffin, 1967; Nudo, 1965) at a time when audiologic services were not readily available or mandatory as a health service for people with disabilities. However, as more recent studies show, in individuals with disabilities from facilities in which audiologic services are available regularly, the incidence of impacted cerumen is no higher than that of the general population (Oyiborhoro, 1993). This is because follow-up cerumen management is instituted when the problem is observed, and the consumer is monitored to ensure that the problem does not become a serious health issue. Personal and ear hygiene may be an issue among consumers with significant cognitive deficits and physical handicaps, but audiologic services including cerumen management should not be an issue.

CERUMEN MANAGEMENT PROCEDURES

Cerumen management in many consumers is definitely more challenging than that in the general population. The choice of procedure must be appropriate for the disability that the consumer presents. At one extreme are consumers who are so spastic that their heads are tilted to the right or left, permanently close to the shoulder. At the other extreme are consumers who are so hypotonic that it is difficult for them to keep and maintain their heads in a suitable position for cerumen removal. In between the two extremes are consumers who often experience sudden jerky and strong involuntary upper body movements (such as those with athetosis) that may make cerumen management rather hazardous if extreme caution is not taken. As previously indicated, the disability presented by a consumer should dictate the appropriate cerumen management technique(s) used.

Cerumen Removal Hazards

Because of the health issues with consumers, it is important to note potential hazards that the clinician is likely to encounter during cerumen removal. This allows more time to prepare so that complications can be better addressed if they arise in the process of cerumen removal.

If cerumen removal instruments are not handled properly, the sudden, involuntary movements often experienced by patients with athetosis can cause scratching of the thin and delicate epithelial lining of the external ear canal, which may cause bleeding. There is also a potential that the tympanic membrane could be perforated. If the irrigating nozzle is not well directed, the water pressure from the irrigation instrument is too high, and if a nonflexible curette is used, serious injury could be inflicted. Thus disposable and more flexible plastic curettes that are likely to cause less trauma in the event of involuntary movement of body parts often encountered with patients with spastic athetosis are commonly used. Examples of plastic and disposable curettes are displayed in Fig. 7.1.

Caution should be exercised when removing cerumen that is firmly attached to or embedded in the wall of the ear canal. If this cerumen is forcefully removed, the upper lining of the canal wall will peel, thereby causing damage to the underlying tissues and bleeding (Serra, 1982). This trauma of cerumen extraction on the auditory canal walls can provoke otitis externa (Ford & Courteney-Harris, 1990).

The use of irrigating fluid at a temperature of 37°C is suggested, because fluctuations in irrigating water temperature in the ear canals can cause vertigo, nausea, and vomiting (Zivic & King, 1993). The external auditory canal is innervated with major cranial nerves. These include the auricular branch of the vagus nerve (cranial nerve X), the auriculotemporal branch of the trigeminal nerve (cranial nerve V), and the posterior auricular branch of the facial nerve (cranial nerve VII). As a result of this network of major cranial nerves, the external auditory canal is quite sensitive, and when it is ordinarily stimulated, it may cause sneezing, coughing, fainting, dizziness, and vomiting. These reactions can be magnified in people with disabilities who present more serious health issues.

Beyond noting of the potential complications, other initial steps include otoscopic examination and obtaining of a medical history.

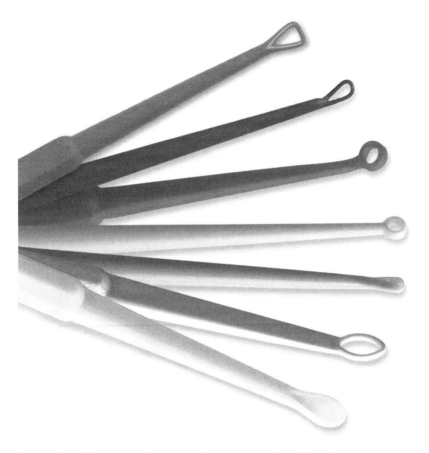

Figure 7.1 Safe curettes. (Reprinted with permission from Bionix.)

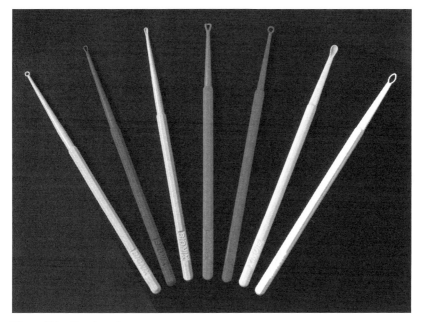

Figure 7.1 Continued

Information from these procedures will determine whether cerumen management is necessary for a consumer.

Otoscopy/Video-Otoscopy

The purpose of otoscopic examination of the ear canal is to evaluate the extent of impaction—whether it is partial or complete and whether the occluding object is indeed cerumen or some other foreign body (such as an insect, a broken head of a Q-tip, or a stone). Another goal of otoscopic examination is to determine whether the external auditory canal is inflamed or whether it is infected, which will necessitate a referral for medical treatment. During otoscopic examination, in addition to gathering evidence for possible contraindications to cerumen removal, the clinician is also able to select cerumen removal techniques that are most appropriate for the consumer and determine whether softening of the cerumen for a few days is necessary before removal.

If a video-otoscope is used, a third party is also able to view the ear canal when the clinician explains the extent of the problem (Fig. 7.2). Usually the consumer is excited about being a part of this process. In most cases the tympanic membrane cannot be visualized when an excessive amount of cerumen is present in the ear canal.

To rule out the possibility of a perforated tympanic membrane, immittance measurement is performed. A flat (type B) tympanogram, high values from the physical volume test, and an inability to obtain and maintain a hermetic seal during immittance are consistent with the possibility of tympanic membrane perforation.

Medical Case History

It is important to examine the medical history of the consumer to determine whether cerumen management is contraindicated, for instance, if (1) the tympanic membrane is perforated or patent pressure equalization (PE) tubes are present, (2) active acquired immune deficiency syndrome (AIDS) is present, and (3) dizziness or any other disease conditions at any portions of the external auditory meatus (pinna, ear canal, and tympanic membrane) or other conditions such as epileptic seizures that may cause complications or put the consumer at risk are present. From the medical case history the clinician determines the most

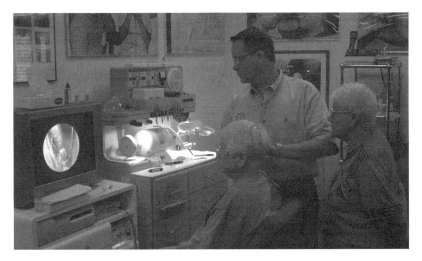

Figure 7.2   Clinican, third party, and consumer view integrity of the tympanic membrane with a video-otoscope. (Photo printed with permission.)

appropriate cerumen management technique for a specific individual with disabilities.

Malignant otitis externa (*Pseudomonas* osteomyelitis) is a serious and life-threatening disease that may develop if the ear canal is irrigated when diabetes mellitus and immunocompromising diseases such as AIDS are present (Ford & Courteney-Harris, 1990; Roeser & Roland, 1992). In nondiabetic, nonimmunocompromised, and healthy individuals, malignant otitis externa is considered a rare occurrence. Malignant otitis externa infection is invasive, and if left untreated, it may lead to osteomyelitis of the skull base with cranial nerve paralysis (Ford & Courteney-Harris, 1990; Zikk, Rapoport, Hamelfarb, 1991). Consumers with diabetes mellitus and immunocompromising disease conditions such as AIDS need a referral for medical treatment.

Cerumen management is done through the use of (1) cerumen extraction instruments such as disposable plastic curettes (see Fig. 7.1), (2) suction, and (3) irrigation or lavage. From our experience with people who have disabilities, irrigation is much faster, more cost effective, and less prone to complications if properly done. Sometimes, when necessary, the three procedures may be used in combination (Ballachanda & Peers, 1992; Graber, 1986). If the cerumen is hard before irrigation, it should be softened by the clinician through application of softening agents of choice. A list of suggested softening agents is displayed in Table 7.2. Softening hard cerumen makes the irrigation procedure much easier and faster and reduces the risk of complications.

CONTRAINDICATIONS TO IRRIGATION

Contraindications to irrigation are similar to some of those noted previously in the section on medical case history. Aural lavage should not be used for cerumen-impacted ears of consumers with the following conditions: (1) perforated tympanic membrane, (2) patent PE tubes, (3) otitis externa, and (4) a history of recent middle ear surgery with a portion of the external auditory canal removed. According to Graber (1986), young children and infants should be excluded because the tympanic membranes of this group may be prone to perforation as a result of lavaging. For children or consumers with PE tubes, there

Table 7.1

Incidence of Excessive/Impacted Cerumen on Different Populations

	Sample Size	Incidence (%)
Children (non–mentally retarded)		
Roche et al. (1978)	224	10
Bricco (1985)	349	10
Adults (non–mentally retarded)		
Lebensohn (1943)	794	2.5
Lebensohn (1943)	3258	8
Perry (1957)	111	17
Hopkinson (1981)	500	4
Foltner (1984)	100	9
Cooper (1985)	587	5
Adolescents (mentally retarded)		
Nudo (1965)	494	36
Fulton & Griffin (1967)	191	28
Brister et al. (1986)	88	22
Crandell & Roeser (in press)	121	28
Geriatric population (non–mentally retarded)		
Mahoney (1987)	242	57
Mahoney (in press)	104	34

From Roeser, R. J., & Roland, P. (1992). What audiologists must know about cerumen management. *American Journal of Audiology, 1*(4), 27–35. (Copyright by the American-Speech-Language-Hearing Association. Reprinted with permission.)

Table 7.2

**Summary of Commercially Available Cerumenolytics and Other Products
Used for Softening Cerumen**

Brand Name	Type	Composition
Audiologists Choice[a]	OTC	Carbamide peroxide (6.5%) and glycerine
Auro Ear Drops	OTC	Carbamide peroxide (6.5%) and glycerine
Bausch & Lomb	OTC	Carbamide peroxide (6.5%) and glycerine
Cerumenex Drops	Rx	Triethanolamine
		Polypeptide
		Oleate condensate
Debrox	OTC	Carbamide peroxide (6.5%) and glycerine
Murine Ear Drops	OTC	Carbamide peroxide (6.5%) and glycerine

Other products for softening cerumen include baby oil, Colace liquid (docusate sodium), hydrogen peroxide (3%), mineral oil, sodium bicarbonate, and virgin olive oil.

[a]Distributed only through audiologists.

OTC, over-the-counter; Rx, prescription.

From Roeser, R. J., & Roland, P. (1992). What audiologists must know about cerumen management. *American Journal of Audiology, 1*(4), 27–35. (Copyright by the American-Speech-Language-Hearing Association. Reprinted with permission.)

is the risk of displacing the tubes (Harkess, 1982). During irrigation, cerumen could be forced through patent PE tubes or a perforated tympanic membrane to the middle ear cavity with the attendant risks of introducing infection (Zivic & King, 1993) into the middle ear cavity. Otitis externa, if present, can be aggravated by irrigation water and pressure.

SOFTENING OF THE CERUMEN

It is our practice to recommend the use of a cerumenolytic agent to soften hard cerumen for 4–5 days before irrigation. Softening the cerumen is important, because it reduces the possibility of using instruments to forcibly extract hard cerumen from the ear canal walls. This can cause a sheering of the skin, damage to the underlying tissues, and pain and bleeding for the consumer.

Over-the-counter (OTC) cerumenolytics that are frequently used include Audiologists Choice, Debrox, and Murine Ear Drops. The chemical compositions of these cerumenolytics are similar: carbamide peroxide (6.5%) and glycerine. Of course, other softening agents such as baby, mineral, or olive oil; Auro Ear Drops; or hydrogen peroxide are also used by some clinicians. Whether Audiologists Choice, Debrox, or Murine Ear Drops are used, the carbamide peroxide chemical element breaks down the cerumen, and the glycerin softens it for removal. If hydrogen peroxide alone is used, there is a tendency for chunks or large, dry particles of cerumen, some of which are still attached to the ear canal walls, to be left behind. Although the effervescence of the hydrogen peroxide breaks down the hard cerumen, it lacks any oily substance to soften it to facilitate the natural self-cleansing process or ease removal by irrigation or lavaging. Before lavaging, consumers, caregivers, or significant others are instructed to apply a few drops (5 to 8 or as indicated in the instructions) of the cerumenolytic agent twice daily for about 4–5 days. The ease of softening of the cerumen depends on the degree of hardness and the depth or quantity of cerumen impaction. If the cerumen is extremely hard and deep in the canal, a few more days of application of the cerumenolytic agent may be required for it to be effective. Some consumers have reported that their hearing became worse after a few days of application of the cerumenolytic agent. This is normal, because in the process of softening of the cerumen some of the matter loosened as a result and closed minute air openings that are sometimes present in a cerumen-impacted ear and allow sound to pass. Once these tiny air pores or ventilation are closed because of the spread of loosened and falling cerumen particles, hearing is significantly affected. However, with the continued use of the softening agent, the air vents open again as the cerumen becomes further softened and loosened.

IRRIGATION OF THE EXTERNAL EAR CANAL

Once the impacted cerumen has been softened, it and other debris can usually be flushed out without difficulties. It is essential that the ear canal be viewed with a video-otoscope or a hand-held otoscope (whichever is available) before lavaging. Also, the integrity of the tympanic membrane must be ascertained before lavaging. Tympanometry should be performed to objectively confirm tympanic membrane integrity. A cerumen-impacted ear canal can be partially opened with the use of a curette to create ventilation to the TM, permitting successful tympanometric assessment (Manning, 1992). Tympanometric findings that yield an usually large canal volume exceeding 1.5 mm suggest the possibility of a perforated tympanic membrane. To remove cerumen, a few items are needed: (1) a Water Pik; (2) a kidney-shaped basin; (3) a plastic apron or cover (water repellant) for the consumer, assistant, and clinician; (4) disposable plastic curettes; (5) paper towels; and (6i) forceps. Water should be kept at body temperature (37°C).

A Water Pik is chosen rather than an ear syringe for two reasons. First, the ear irrigator that attaches to the Water Pik is long and more flexible, and the nozzle is easier to direct to the roof of the ear canal walls. Second, the irrigator can provide a constant stream of water at slow or fast pulsating pressure that can be controlled. On the other hand, the pressure produced by an ear syringe is more variable, the instrument is relatively large, and it is fairly difficult to match the flexibility offered by an ear irrigator, especially when one is performing the procedure on a consumer with athetosis or one who is very spastic with his or her head permanently tilted close to the shoulder, leaving little or no room in which to work. As a result of the attributes stated above, a Water Pik is recommended for use (Larsen, 1976; Roeser & Roland, 1983). The procedure is explained to the consumer and the accompanying caregiver or family member. Some consumers may be unable to comprehend the instructions given because of the degree of mental deficiency or, if they do understand, are unable to follow commands because of neuromotor deficits.

Once the consumer is comfortably seated, the Water Pik is filled with lukewarm water or body temperature water kept at 37°C. The use of cold or hot water to lavage the ear canal can stimulate the semicircular canals, which may provoke the vestibular reflex, causing dizziness, nausea, and vomiting (Roeser & Roland, 1992; Zivic & King, 1993). The irrigating nozzle is placed in the ear canal while the pinna is pulled upward and backward to straighten the canal. The stream of water from the irrigation nozzle is directed to the posterior walls of the roof of the ear canal to the right and then to the left until sufficient pressure has built up behind the cerumen plug to flush it out. Unlike with an ear syringe, it is easy to pull out the nozzle if the consumer is experiencing tremors. It is not advisable to direct the stream of water at the cerumen for two reasons. First, the pressure can force the cerumen deeper into the canal. Second, if the cerumen was already very loose, the tympanic membrane may be exposed to a direct hit from the water stream. This can cause serious damage. Therefore the water stream is directed at the roof of the canal in a steady state with the goal of gaining access of flow behind the cerumen and debris. Once this is achieved, the cerumen is flushed out. The ear canal is checked periodically with a video-otoscope or hand-held otoscope to determine the effectiveness of the lavaging process. Consumers are always excited to see the "inside" of their ears while the procedure is in progress. Small chunks of cerumen can be removed, with a disposable plastic curette. The use of plastic curettes rather than the metallic type is preferable. If there is a sudden jerk or uncontrolled body movements by the consumer while lavaging is in progress, the risk of physical injury is less severe with use of disposable plastic curettes.

Lavaging continues until the tympanic membrane becomes visible. The water stream, pressure, and flow should be reduced at this time to avoid accidental physical insult to the tympanic membrane. The ear canal is examined again with an otoscope to ensure that the tympanic membrane is intact. Again, this can be achieved objectively by performing tympanometry. The ear canal should be checked to ensure that there is no bleeding and the canal is free of excessive cerumen and debris. The ear canal is then dried by an applicator moistened with 70% isopropyl alcohol. The clinician must ensure that there is no bleeding before alcohol solution is applied.

REFERENCES

Adams, G., Boies, L., & Papparella, M. (1978). *Fundamentals of Otolaryngology.* Philadelphia: WB Saunders.

Ballachanda, B. B., & Peers, C. J. (1992, February). Cerumen management: Instruments and procedures. *ASHA, 34,* 43–46.

Bricco, E. (1985). Impacted cerumen as a reason for failure in hearing; Conservation programs. *Journal of School Health, 55,* 240–241.

Brister, F., Fullwood, H. L., Ripp, T., & Blodgett, C. (1986). Prevalence of occlusion due to impacted cerumen among mentally retarded adolescents. *American Journal of Mental Deficiency, 91,* 302–304.

Crandell, C. C., & Roeser, R. J. (1993). Incidence of excessive/impacted cerumen in mentally retarded individuals. *American Journal of Mental Retardation, 97,* 568–574.

Ford, G. R., & Courteney-Harris, R. G. (1990). Another hazard of ear syringing: Malignant external otitis. *The Journal of Laryngology and Otology, 104,* 709–710.

Fulton, R., & Griffin, C. (1967). Audiological-otological considerations with the mentally retarded. *Mental Retardation, 5*(3), 26–31.

Graber, R. F. (1986). Removing impacted cerumen. *Patient Care, 20,* 151–153.

Harkess, C. K. (1982, January–February). Clearing the occluded canal. *Pediatric Nurse,* 23–25.

Kirkwood, D. H. (1993). The cerumen management debated: Whose responsibility is it? *The Hearing Journal, 46,* 13–22.

Larsen, G. (1976). Removing cerumen with a Water Pik. *American Journal of Nursing, 76,* 264–265.

Manning, R. (1992). *Cerumen management.* Lexington, KY: Eastern Kentucky Speech and Hearing Clinic.

Northern, J., & Downs, M. (1984). *Hearing in children* (3rd ed.). Baltimore: William & Wilkins.

Nudo, L. (1965). Comparison by age of audiological and otological findings in a state residential institution for the mentally retarded: A preliminary report. In Loyd, L., & Frisina, R. (Eds.). *Audiological assessment of the mentally retarded: Proceedings of national conference.* Parsons, KS: Parsons State Hospital and Training Center.

Oyiborhoro, J. M. A. (1993, April). *Impacted cerumen in cerebral palsy population.* Paper presented to The American Academy of Audiology, Phoenix, Arizona.

Roeser, R. J., & Roland, P. (1992). What audiologists must know about cerumen management. *American Journal of Audiology, 1,* 27–35.

Ruby, R. F. (1986). Conductive hearing loss in the elderly. *Journal of Otolaryngology, 15,* 245–247.

Serra, A. (1982). Ear syringing. *Nursing Mirror, 155,* 10–12.

Stone, M., & Fulghum, R. S. (1984). Bactericidal activity of wet cerumen. *Annals of Otology, Rhinology, and Laryngology, 93,* 183–186.

Zikk, D., Rapoport, Y., & Hamelfarb, M. Z. (1991). Invasive external otitis after removal of impacted cerumen by irrigation. *New England Journal of Medicine, 325,* 969–970.

Zivic, R. C., & King, S. (1993). Cerumen impaction management for clients of all ages. *Nurse Practitioner, 18,* 29–37.

SELECTED READINGS

Baily, B. J. (1983). Impacted ear wax and water pick instrument. *Journal of Medicine, 250,* 1456.

Seiler, E. R. (1980). Ear syringing. *British Medical Journal, 280,* 1273.

PART II

Alternative Communication, Amplification, and Counseling

CHAPTER 8

Amplification and Assistive Technology

Kenneth C. Pugh, Ph.D.
Division of Speech Pathology and Audiology
John A. Burns School of Medicine
University of Hawaii at Manoa
Honolulu, HA

Amplification
> Hearing Instrument Styles
> Hearing Aid Circuits
> Selection, Fitting, and Verification of Hearing
>   Instruments
> Troubleshooting Hearing Instruments
> Hearing Instruments versus Assistive Technology

Assistive Technology
> Enhancing Listening Ability
> Capitalizing on Modalities Other Than Hearing
> Selecting Assistive Technology

Trends in Amplification and Assistive Technology
Conclusions
Acknowledgments
References

This chapter provides information on amplification and assistive technology. The focus is on currently available amplification in the form of hearing instruments and assistive technology that can be used to either enhance listening ability or capitalize on modalities other than hearing.

Selection, fitting guidelines, and the rationale for providing these systems as a component of the rehabilitation process are included.

AMPLIFICATION

Rehabilitative intervention used to assist persons with sensory disability resulting from hearing impairment typically occurs through the provision of amplification. The principle role of amplification in the form of hearing instruments (hearing aids) is to increase sounds to levels such that persons with hearing impairment can both detect and make use of the auditory signals. The use of hearing instruments dates back to the nineteenth century, when amplification was initially achieved by cupping the hand behind the ear—a practice still used today—or with different types of ear horns and ear trumpets (Berger, 1984; Lybarger, 1988). Since that time, successive advancements have led to the production of carbon hearing instruments, vacuum tube hearing instruments, transistor hearing instruments, and integrated circuit hearing instruments (Dillon, 2001; Vonlanthen, 2000). Each stage of development is sequential, which means that smaller and smaller hearing instruments are being produced to the point where the amplification device could be worn at ear level or within the ear canal.

Hearing Instrument Styles

Existing amplification options include hearing aid styles such as body style, behind the ear (BTE), in the ear (ITE), in the canal (ITC), and completely in the canal (CIC) instruments. Body style devices represent an older form of electronic hearing instrument and serve as a means of amplification when nothing else will provide enough power. A receiver is connected to the hearing aid with a cord, and this hearing aid is usually worn in a shirt pocket or clipped to clothing. Body style hearing aids provide amplification for extremely severe hearing loss, for a bedridden patient, or for an individual who may have difficulty using the controls of a smaller ear level hearing instrument because of reduced dexterity. However, body style hearing instruments are considered cosmetically less appealing and cumbersome because of their large size and cords, and as a result, this hearing instrument is not often used.

A BTE-style hearing instrument is shown in Fig. 8.1. As the name implies, components of the hearing instrument are held in the casing positioned behind the ear, and sound travels through the hearing instrument into an earmold and finally into the ear canal. The BTE-style hearing instrument can be used by people of all ages with mild to profound hearing loss. Because of the growth changes that occur in young children, BTE-style hearing instruments are often selected as the amplification devices of choice when they present with hearing impairment.

The BTE-style hearing instrument is more visible than other hearing aids worn at ear level but provides benefits that smaller styles do not offer. For example, the biggest advantage to the BTE hearing aid is the ability to use this hearing instrument with telecoil capability and direct audio input. The telecoil picks up electromagnetic signals, such as those from telephones, and converts them into an electrical signal that is amplified by the hearing instrument. With direct audio input (DAI), the BTE hearing aid can be attached to a hardwire or wireless audio "boot," which links the hearing instrument to either a personal or sound field frequency-modulated (FM) amplification system. The DAI allows the hearing aid microphone to remain on while the FM signal is picked up. The DAI also can be connected to a television, stereo, tape recorder, or personal radio. These components are addressed further in the section on assistive technology.

The ITE-style hearing instrument (Fig. 8.2) fits in the concha and outer ear cavity and is used to assist those with mild to severe hearing impairments. The ITE-style hearing instrument can provide more amplification than canal hearing aid styles, and individuals who do or do not need glasses can use this style comfortably. In addition, those who produce little to moderate amounts of cerumen (earwax) may find this hearing aid style suitable for their needs. Because it is worn within the ear canal, it is more cosmetically appealing than larger hearing aid styles, and individuals with good family support can still choose this model if their family helps them change the tiny battery.

The ITC-style hearing instrument (Fig. 8.3) is worn within the ear canal and can be used for mild to moderate hearing loss. It is not able to provide as much amplification as larger hearing aid styles. However,

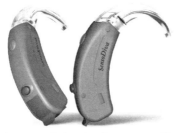

Figure 8.1   A behind-the-ear–style hearing instrument. (Reprinted with permission from Widex Hearing Aid Company, Inc.)

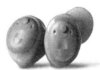

Figure 8.2   An in-the-ear–style hearing instrument. (Reprinted with permission from Widex Hearing Aid Compay, Inc.)

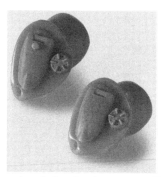

Figure 8.3   An in-the-canal–style hearing instrument. (Reprinted with permission from Phonak Hearing Instruments.)

individuals with poor manual dexterity or arthritis may experience slight difficulty when manipulating the user controls (e.g., battery door, volume controls, and insertion and removal of the hearing instrument).

Finally, the CIC-style hearing instrument (Fig. 8.4) is worn deeply within the external ear canal and is used for mild to moderate hearing loss. Because the CIC-style hearing instrument is positioned completely within the ear canal, it is cosmetically appealing and often the amplification style of choice for many persons with hearing loss. Key to the successful use of this instrument is proper insertion and removal. A built-in insertion and removal line that extends from many CIC-style hearing instruments is principally how this task is accomplished (Fig. 8.5). Persons with disabilities who experience poor vision and dexterity or arthritis may also encounter difficulty when using the CIC-style hearing instrument.

HEARING AID CIRCUITS

Besides choosing a hearing aid style that best suits the person with hearing impairment, there are also different types of integrated circuitry that require consideration: analog, digitally programmable analog, and fully digital. It is important to note that any of these circuitry types can be included within any hearing instrument style (i.e., BTE, ITE, ITC, and CIC), which greatly influences the overall costs. Analog hearing aids use conventional integrated circuitry for signal processing. In other words, analog hearing instruments have a microphone that picks up continuously varying sounds in the environment, converts the sounds into an electrical signal, and amplifies the electrical signal, which is transduced via the receiver back to acoustic sounds to fit the needs of the hearing aid user. This hearing aid circuit is considered linear, because it amplifies all sounds to the capable limits of the device, no matter how loud the incoming sounds are. Most analog hearing instruments are suitable for patients who need basic amplification at the lowest price. Patients who have difficulty adjusting to new technology and who do not spend time in various environments with many people may find this type of circuitry adequate.

Digitally programmable analog (hybrid) circuitry functions in the same fashion as analog circuitry; however, the parameters in which the

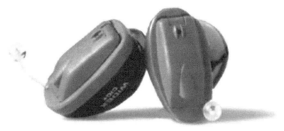

Figure 8.4   A completely-in-the-canel–style hearing instrument. (Reprinted with permission from Widex Hearing Aid Company, Inc.)

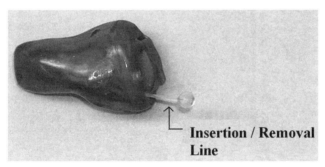

Figure 8.5   Illustration of an insertion and removal line on a completely-in-the-canal–style hearing instrument.

signals are processed are controlled digitally. That is, the integrated circuitry makes use of a cable connection from the hearing instrument to a personal computer or special programming equipment, which allows the hearing health care practitioner to determine the boundaries in which the hearing aid amplifies sounds. The analog parameters can be altered and sound quality comparisons can be determined in terms of speech understanding and noise as well as in quiet conditions. Instead of linear amplification, digitally programmable analog circuitry uses compression, a means of providing amplification by boosting soft sounds to audible levels and suppressing loud sounds to levels that are more comfortable and compatible with the person's hearing loss.

Fully digital hearing instruments are the most advanced and most expensive types of integrated circuitry. Incoming sounds are converted into binary numbers, which are then analyzed and manipulated via a set of rules (algorithms) programmed into the computer chip that controls the hearing instrument. Fully digital circuitry also makes use of compression and a cable connection from the hearing instrument to a personal computer or special programming equipment, which allows the hearing health care practitioner to manipulate the settings. Thus digital hearing aid circuitry has much more flexibility for processing sounds (e.g., use of preprogrammed settings that can be used when a person moves from quiet environments to noisy environments) than analog and strictly bound hybrid integrated circuits. Patients who do not have difficulty adjusting to new technology and who spend time in various environments will find this type of circuitry appropriate.

SELECTION, FITTING, AND VERIFICATION OF HEARING INSTRUMENTS

Selection and fitting of hearing instruments often starts by determining whether the person is a candidate for amplification. Definitive candidacy requirements can vary from one hearing health care professional to another, yet most individuals are considered candidates when their hearing impairment affects the audiometric frequency range that is critical for clear understanding of speech (i.e., 1–4 kHz). In pediatric patients or in patients with unreliable behavioral responses during routine audiometric tests, candidacy can be determined via auditory brainstem response tests (Dalzell et al., 2000; Lin, Shu, Chang, & Bruna, 2002; Mason & Herrmann, 1998; Sakai, Watanabe, & Kaga, 2002). The decision for hearing instrument use can be based on these audiometric data as well as on equally important nonaudiometric components such as age, speech and language development, existence of other medical conditions, family and ancillary support, motivation level, or special needs. From a more subjective point of view, candidacy for hearing aid use is highly probable when the person with hearing difficulty reports that others are constantly mumbling during conversations, has the ability to hear and not fully understand what others are saying, has a longstanding history of hearing difficulty across various environments, or is constantly turning up the volume on the television or radio to the point at which other family members complain. Each of these nonaudiometric components can greatly influence hearing instrument use or the amount of additional habilitation or rehabilitation involved.

Once a person has undergone an audiometric evaluation, it is often recommended that the person obtain medical clearance for hearing aid use. Guidelines set forth by the U.S. Food and Drug Administration indicate that all children require written medical clearance by a physician and/otorhinolaryngologist (ear-nose-and-throat specialist) for hearing instrument use, and this clearance should be obtained within 6 months prior to the date of sale of the hearing instrument or instruments. However, individuals 18 years of age and older may either obtain medical clearance or sign a waiver in lieu of obtaining medical clearance. When this occurs and the person has been determined as a candidate for amplification, the hearing instrument fitting process ensues. In this process, the hearing health care professional will work with the client to select hearing instrument style and integrated circuitry, gain, frequency response, and maximum power output characteristics. The term *gain* refers to the difference in loudness (measured in decibel sound pressure level [dB SPL]) between the sound going into the hearing instrument and the sound leaving the hearing instrument. For instance, if the sound going into the hearing instrument is 45 dB SPL and the sound leaving the hearing instrument is 75 dB SPL, then the hearing instrument in this case has 30 dB of gain. When gain is plotted as a function of frequency (measured in Hz), it creates a distribution across different sounds that are amplified by the device, otherwise known as the frequency response (Lucks-Mendel, Danhauer, & Singh, 1999). Finally, maximum power output refers to a level beyond that which the hearing instrument cannot amplify and serves as a means of protecting the hearing instrument user from uncomfortably loud sounds.

The hearing instrument selection process usually occurs *before* the actual hearing aid fitting session itself; hence, focus is placed on preselecting the necessary gain and maximum power output values. Gain and maximum power output values rely heavily on computer-based prescriptive hearing instrument fitting formulas—a blueprint that links a person's hearing-impairment to certain amplification characteristics. Examples of common prescription-based hearing instrument fitting formulas are shown in Table 8.1. These prescription-based fitting formulas are often selected according to audiometric hearing thresholds, suprathreshold perception of loudness, and listening situations in which the hearing instruments will be worn. For extended reviews of prescriptive hearing instrument fitting formulas, the interested reader is directed to Dillon (2001) and Valente (2002a, 2002b).

To document the adequacy of the hearing instrument after the fitting process has occurred, it is essential to verify the hearing aid fitting using both objective and subjective measures. Perhaps the most popular objective means of hearing aid verification is real ear measurements—determining the functional properties of the hearing instrument while the user is wearing the hearing instrument. Advances in measuring hearing aid performance in this manner have led to the development of commercially available equipment and probe tube microphone instrumentation (Mueller, Hawkins, & Northern, 1992). This allows measurement of the response of the hearing instrument while it is in the person's ear at quiet, mid, and high intensity levels. Conversely, a subjective method used to verify hearing instrument performance is obtaining behavioral functional gain, which involves measuring the difference between speech perception ability with (aided) versus without (unaided) hearing instruments. As an alternative to behavioral functional gain measures, an equally important subjective process used to verify hearing instrument performance is obtaining a self-report of benefit from the hearing aid user. These hearing aid benefit measures serve to quantify how hearing aid use affects the fulfillment of life activities with specific emphasis on daily communication (McCarthy, 1997). Among the more common self-assessment scales used to measure hearing aid benefit and how hearing impairment affects the social and emotional aspects of

Table 8.1

Examples of Prescription-Based Hearing Instrument Fitting Formulas

DSL [i/o]	Desired Sensation Level Input-Output for Compression Amplification (Cornelisse, Seewald, & Jamieson, 1955)
FIG6	Figure 6 Fitting Procedure (Killion & Fikret-Pasa, 1993)
IHAFF	Indenpendent Hearing Aid Fitting Forum Loudness Scaling Procedure (Cox, 1995; Valente & Van Vliet, 1997)
LGOB	Loudness Growth in Half-Octave Bands (Allen, Hall, & Jeng, 1990)
NAL	National Acoustic Laboratories Fitting Procedure Byrne & Tonisson, 1976)
NAL-NL1	National Acoustic Laboratories, Nonlinear, Version 1 (Dillon, 1999)
POGO	Prescription of Gain and Output (McCandless & Lyregaard, 1983)

hearing loss are the Abbreviated Profile of Hearing Aid Benefit (APHAB) and the Hearing Handicap Inventory for the Elderly (HHIE).

The APHAB, which is a condensed version of the 64-item Profile of Hearing Aid Benefit (PHAB) (Cox & Rivera, 1992), is a standardized 24-item self-assessment tool designed to assess auditory performance with and without hearing aids across various listening environments (Cox & Alexander, 1995). The 24 questions are divided into four subscales (Ease of Communication [EC], Background Noise [BN], Reverberation [RV], and Aversiveness of Sounds [AV]), consisting of six questions each. Individuals are instructed to answer according to a seven-point response scale with assigned percentages (i.e., always, 99%; almost always, 87%; generally, 75%; half the time, 50%; occasionally, 25%; seldom, 12%; never, 1%) to each component. All items on the APHAB are answered twice, once for "without the hearing aid" and again for "with the hearing aid."

The HHIE (Ventry & Weinstein, 1982) is a 25-question self-assessment tool designed to assess the effects of hearing impairment on the emotional and social adjustment of adults older than age 65 years. There is also a version of this inventory that can be used for adults younger than age 65 years, the Hearing Handicap Inventory for Adults (HHIA) (Newman, Weinstein, Jacobson, & Hug, 1990). The HHIE/A has a 13-item subscale that explores the emotional consequences of hearing impairment and a 12-item subscale that explores both social and situational effects of hearing impairment. Individuals are instructed to answer "Yes," "Sometimes," or "No" for each item. Responses are allocated 4, 2, and 0 points, respectively, and scores for each subscale are combined to produce a total score. The minimum possible score that can be obtained on the HHIE/A is 0, whereas the maximum possible score that can be obtained on the HHIE/A is 100. Higher scores indicate increased emotional, social, and situational difficulties associated with hearing impairment. With the APHAB and the HHIE/A, verification of the amount of hearing aid benefit is demonstrated by the difference in scores before and after hearing aid fitting (Humes, Halling, & Coughlin, 1996).

TROUBLESHOOTING HEARING INSTRUMENTS

Over the course of hearing instrument use, various circumstances under which the hearing aid will malfunction and require routine checks will be seen. The most straightforward way to determine whether the hearing instrument has malfunctioned is to use a troubleshooting sequence or a series of steps to follow that allows hearing instrument users to ascertain why their hearing instrument is not working properly. The initial step to determine a faulty hearing instrument is a general cleaning of the device. During this process a soft cloth can be used to remove dirt, moisture, or cerumen from all surface areas. Clogs in the earmold should be cleaned using the earmold tubing blower. After the general cleaning, another step is for the user to physically inspect the hearing instrument to determine whether the casing has any cracks or broken parts. For instance, cracks in the BTE hearing aid tubing or cracks and broken parts in the shell casing may require an immediate visit to the hearing health care professional for repair.

A next step in the troubleshooting process is determining that the battery is properly placed within the hearing instrument. As with all batteries, these have both a positive and a negative side, and their correct placement within the hearing instrument is usually determined by either a plus (+) or minus (−) sign shown on the battery door. This circumstance serves as both an advantage and a disadvantage, because only with good vision or under adequate magnification can this "+" or "−" sign be seen. To ease some of the difficulties that arise with correct battery placement, battery dispensers are available. A battery dispenser is a relatively new device that simplifies the process by allowing the user to transfer the battery directly from the packaging into the hearing instrument. This reduces the chances of dropping and losing the battery during the process.

Two other items equally important to correct battery placement are making sure that the battery contacts inside the hearing instrument are clean and free of corrosive materials and that the correct size battery is being used. Table 8.2 provides information on battery sizes for each hearing instrument style (i.e., BTE, ITE, ITC, and CIC); these sizes have color-coded tabs for easy identification when they are purchased. Most hearing aid batteries are known as Zinc-Air, or are constructed to use air from outside the battery as the activating agent once the color-coded tab is removed. Although most Zinc-Air batteries produce 1.3 to 1.5 V, replacing the color-coded tab when the battery is not in use will not extend the battery life. Battery life fluctuates according to conditions such as the number of hours each day the hearing instrument is being used, the volume control settings while the hearing instrument is in use,

Table 8.2

Available Zinc-Air Battery Sizes for Hearing Instruments

Battery size	Hearing instrument style	Color coded tab
675	BTE	Blue
13	BTE or ITE	Orange
312	ITE or ITC	Brown
10 (10A)	ITC or CIC	Yellow
5 (5A)	CIC	Red

the size of the battery, and the type of integrated circuitry within the hearing instrument.

Once the hearing instrument has been cleaned, is determined to be free from any cracks and breaks, and has an adequately charged battery that is properly inserted, the final step is a listening check. A person who does not have any hearing difficulty should perform the listening check, and a hearing aid stethoscope (Fig. 8.6) should be used to conduct this component of the troubleshooting process. By turning on and attaching the hearing instrument to the hearing aid stethoscope, the listener can determine the clarity of sounds such as /u/ /i/, /s/, /sh/, /m/, and /n/. While adjustments are made to the volume, an inventory of any intermittence, static, unexplained feedback, or interference is also made while the person talks at various loudness levels. Unwanted sounds (e.g., humming or static) determined during the process would probably require further troubleshooting or repair. In addition to these suggestions, a regularly scheduled maintenance plan with the hearing health care professional should allow for more exhaustive evaluation and resolution of any hearing aid malfunction.

HEARING INSTRUMENTS VERSUS ASSISTIVE TECHNOLOGY

Amplification in the form of hearing instruments is considered the primary option for many individuals who are hearing-impaired; however, they are not designed to address every listener's needs. The rapid development of hearing instrument technology over the past several years has made it possible to produce higher fidelity instruments, yet the biggest limitation often reported among hearing aid users is the inability to clearly comprehend the spoken message in the presence of competing noise or when the listener is not in close proximity to the person speaking (Flexer, 1999; Franks & Beckmann, 1985).

Despite miniaturization of hearing instruments (the trend toward increasingly smaller hearing instruments), large numbers of persons with hearing impairment choose not to use them. An examination of the literature concerning the reasons for this discrepancy between the numbers of individuals in the United States with hearing loss who require hearing aid use and those who actually use hearing aids reveals several factors. These factors include social stigma, instrument reliability,

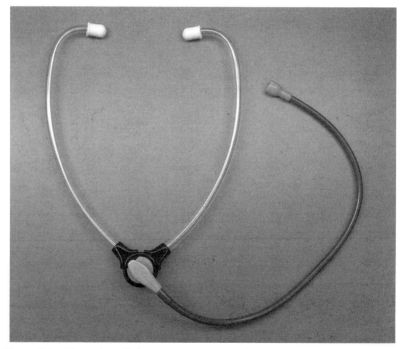

Figure 8.6   Illustration of a hearing instrument stethoscope used for a listening check.

performance quality, sales practices of hearing health care practitioners, perception of hearing loss, and cost of the hearing instruments (Franks & Beckmann, 1985; Kochkin, 1992, 1993, 1998; Mark, 2000). These conditions explain why assistive technology has become an increasingly feasible alternative for persons with (and without) hearing impairment.

ASSISTIVE TECHNOLOGY

The Technology-Related Assistance for Individuals with Disabilities Act of 1988 (U.S. Public Law 100-407), otherwise known as the Tech Act, defines assistive technology as "any item, piece of equipment or product system, whether acquired commercially off the shelf, modified or customized, that is used to increase or improve functional capabilities of individuals with disabilities." The Tech Act provides funding to develop statewide, consumer-responsive information and training programs designed to meet the assistive technology needs of individuals with disabilities. Just as with hearing instruments, assistive technology serves to increase independence of persons with disabilities and can further improve communicative functioning, because benefits are obtained by either enhancing listening ability or by capitalizing on modalities other than hearing. As the number of persons in need of assistive technology has grown, the industry that designs, produces, and markets these devices has grown substantially as well.

ENHANCING LISTENING ABILITY

Assistive technology in the form of an FM amplification system can be used to overcome limitations imposed by persons with and without hearing impairment. In the United States, FM amplification systems are sanctioned by the Federal Communications Commission, a United States government agency that regulates radiofrequency usage to broadcast on two designated radio frequency bands: 72–76 MHz and 216–217 MHz. The FM amplification system can transmit sounds anywhere from 30 to 200 feet. This provides users of this technology with the ability to comprehend spoken messages in the presence of competing noise, even when the listener is not in close proximity to the person speaking.

Although a number of different commercial FM amplification systems are available, they usually consist of a basic set of components: a microphone, a transmitter, and a receiver. The personal FM receiver worn by the listener must be set to the same channel and radiofrequency as the microphone/transmitter worn by the person speaking. The microphone is offered in several styles, including lavaliere, lapel, and boom. Lavaliere microphones are small and are usually positioned around the neck of the person speaking. Lapel microphones are typically clipped to a pocket, tie, or lapel of the person speaking, and the microphone should be placed approximately 6 inches away from the person's mouth. Jewelry or other loose items that could rub or bump against the microphone should be removed before use. Another option is the boom microphone that is worn on the head, secured by a headband. The transmitter is worn by the person speaking and is small enough to be placed in a pocket. The receiver is typically worn by the listener in a chest harness or on a belt with individual FM systems.

Two types of FM amplification systems are commonly used: individual FM systems and sound-field FM systems. Individual amplification systems can be further grouped into two categories: a self-contained system and a personal FM system. The difference between these two types of individual systems depends on how the sound is delivered to the listener's ears. A self-contained amplification system, also known as an auditory trainer, typically delivers sound through earphones. A self-contained auditory trainer amplification system is shown in Fig. 8.7. Sounds are channeled from the environment to the receiver control box and into the headphones. The receiver unit contains environmental microphones and volume control dials, allowing the user to control the level of amplification. If the listener has a hearing loss and wears hearing aids, then he or she is required to remove them when using this system. Most individuals who use the self-contained system have severe to profound hearing impairments; however, individuals with lesser degrees of hearing loss and no hearing aids can benefit from using an auditory trainer as well (Flexer, 1999).

A personal FM amplification system is similar to the auditory trainer. The only difference is that this system is coupled with a person's own hearing aid. A personal FM amplification system is shown in Fig. 8.8. Sounds are channeled from the hearing aid through the FM system, making this system dependent on the integrity of hearing instrument

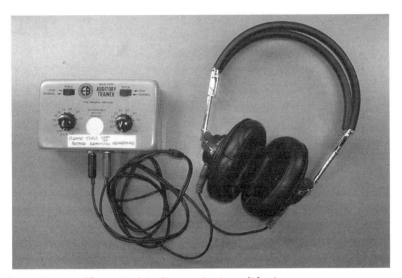

Figure 8.7   A self-contained (auditory trainer) amplification system.

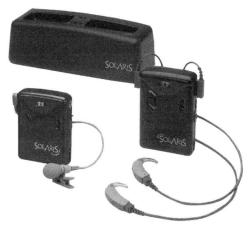

Figure 8.8   A personal FM amplification system with charger. (Reprinted with permission from Phonic Ear, Inc.)

function. Coupling options for personal FM amplification systems include neckloop, silhouette, and DAI. Each coupling arrangement has advantages and disadvantages, and these differences should be considered when the clinician chooses an option for the individual with hearing impairment. The neckloop coupling option is a wire or loop that is worn loosely around the listener's neck and is attached to the FM receiver. The wire receives the electrical signal and generates an electromagnetic field that is picked up by the person's hearing aid when the aid is set to the telecoil "T" setting. An advantage to using the neckloop fitting is that there are no connecting wires between the receiver and the hearing aid. Also, the neckloop can be worn under clothes, reducing the cosmetic concern associated with use of amplification devices. Potential drawbacks with the neckloop arrangement are increased equipment noise with this coupling option and effects on signal strength with changes in head positioning.

As mentioned earlier, the biggest advantage to use of the BTE hearing instrument is its DAI coupling to a personal FM system capability. With the DAI coupling option, mechanical interfaces have been developed to allow users to combine their BTEs with a personal or sound-field FM amplification system. The electrical signal from an FM receiver is directed into the hearing aid through an audio "shoe" or "boot." These boots come in various shapes and must be fitted snugly on the hearing aid to minimize signal disruption. Figure 8.9 illustrates the coupling of a BTE hearing instrument to a receiver of a wireless FM system. This arrangement allows wireless connection capability with several different BTE hearing instruments currently available on the market. Key to its efficient use is the presence on the hearing aid of a special DAI feature that allows accommodation of the boot; this feature is available on many BTE hearing instruments and on a limited number of ITE hearing instruments.

Unlike individual FM amplification systems, sound-field FM systems allow everyone within an entire area, such as a classroom setting, to benefit from amplification. A sound-field FM amplification system is shown in Fig. 8.10. In this case there is no need for the microphone/transmitter and receiver to be set to the same channel. Instead, the speech signal delivered into the microphone/transmitter by the person speaking is amplified and routed to loudspeakers placed around the room. The use of a wireless microphone by the person speaking allows additional mobility. With sound-field FM amplification, the speaker's

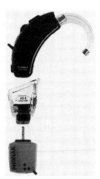

Figure 8.9   A behind-the-ear–style hearing instrument coupled with an audio "shoe" and a wireless FM receiver. (Reprinted with permission from Phonak Ear, Inc.)

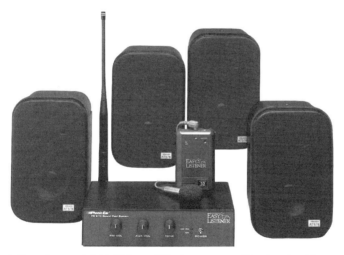

Figure 8.10   A sound-field FM amplification system. (Reprinted with permission from Phonic Ear, Inc.)

voice can be raised at least 10–15 dB above the surrounding ambient noise, improving the signal-to-noise ratio and enabling greater understanding of what is being said (Crandell, Smaldino, & Flexer, 1995).

Battery chargers also need to be considered when FM amplification systems are used. Optimal function is obtained when the batteries for both the FM transmitter and the FM receiver are charged regularly. The charging units are plugged into a standard wall socket, and the time required for charging will vary from 8 to 12 hours. Battery chargers are available in three main types: case chargers, modular chargers, and wall chargers. Case chargers include spaces for 12 charging units. Modular chargers are 2-pocket chargers but can be expanded by adding up to 12 more pockets. Wall types allow for charging both transmitter and receiver pairs.

Induction loop amplification systems are another form of assistive technology that can be used to overcome limitations imposed by less than ideal listening conditions for persons with and without hearing impairment. The properties of induction loop amplification are similar to those of a public address system. Speech directed into a microphone is amplified and fed into a wire that is routed around a designated area of space. The area of space creates a looped field and may be as limited as the immediate circumference around an individual or as large as a seating section in an auditorium, church, or theater. The system works by transducing the acoustic properties from speech spoken into the microphone to electromagnetic energy conducted through the wire. Persons sitting within the looped field can receive sound naturally through the loudspeakers in the environment or via the electromagnetic signal by wearing amplification that is sensitive to magnetic field changes, such as a T-switch on a hearing instrument or personal FM receiver.

Infrared systems are a wireless type of assistive technology used to transmit signals by invisible light waves to the listener. The system consists of a transmitter, called an emitter, and a receiver that has an "eye" (diode) on it. For the system to function properly, the diode picks up the light waves from the emitter and converts them to sound. Any number of receivers can be used with the emitter, as long as each diode is within the line of sight of the emitter (Crandell et al., 1995). A factor that can inhibit the performance of an infrared system is the amount of interference caused by lighting within the room as well as natural sunlight. Direct sunlight contains a large amount of infrared light and can block the signal if the sunlight shines directly on the receiver diode.

Other types of assistive technology can be used to enhance the speaker-to-listener conduit and are suitable for most clients regardless of their hearing ability. They include wake-up alarms and amplified cordless, cell, digital, and hard-wired telephones. With most standard telephones, the user is not able to change the volume level. When additional amplification is necessary, an amplified telephone (Fig. 8.11) can allow for a range of 30 to 50 dB of gain. Amplified phones have additional features such as large dialing buttons, moderately sized LCD screens, and strobe ring signalers, making it easier for use when numbers are dialed or emitting flashing lights when the telephone rings.

Capitalizing on Modalities Other Than Hearing

Assistive communication devices that do not emphasize listening ability include telecommunication devices for the deaf (TDD), computerized speech recognition programs, closed caption decoders, and visual alerting devices. These types of assistive technology go as far back as the 1960s, when telephone modems were first linked with telephone type-writers (TTYs), enabling persons with hearing impairment to converse via phone lines by typing conversations back and forth (Rothstein & Everson, 1995). Today, computerized speech recognition systems, desktop computers, and laptop computers have the ability to provide audio trans-mission or display textual versions of speech in real time. Because the computerized speech recognition system is configured as a best fit of a linguistic parse, the textual on-screen presentation may differ from the speaker's actual utterances, depending on factors of dialect, format frequencies, and the actual computer program itself (Molnar et al., 2000; Sutton, 1997). For these reasons, there may be situations in which the individual and his or her speaking partner may need to repair the conversation on occasion.

Alerting devices display a visual or tactile signal when a sound occurs. The alerting system may be a strobe light, conventional light, or flashing light. If vision is poor, vibrating pages or a service dog can alert the client. Although several organizations provide these animals, Canine Companions for Independence (www.caninecompanions.org) is a 501(c)(3) nonprofit organization that serves to enhance the lives of

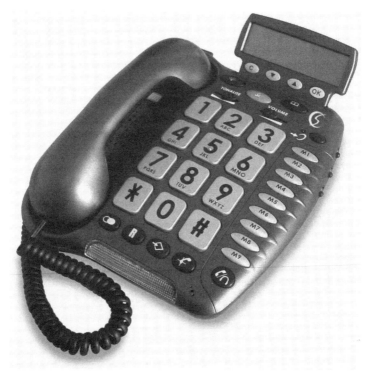

Figure 8.11   Illustration of an amplified telephone. (Reprinted with permission from HITEC Group International, Inc.)

people with disabilities by providing highly trained assistance dogs and ongoing support to ensure quality partnerships. Founded in 1975, Canine Companions for Independence pioneered the concept of training dogs to assist people with physical disabilities. An assistance dog is trained to help its owner deal with physical obstacles in daily life as well as signal its owner to environmental sounds such as smoke alarms, telephones, doorbells, and clock alarms. People with physical or developmental disabilities who can demonstrate that a trained assistance dog will enhance their independence or their quality of life are eligible to apply at regional centers throughout the United States. Also eligible are professionals working for organizations that provide physical or mental health care to clients who could benefit, and there is usually no charge for the dog.

SELECTING ASSISTIVE TECHNOLOGY

Selection of assistive technology often occurs by conducting a functional assessment of the potential user's abilities. Hearing impairment (if any) along with limitations in cognitive or physical abilities should be documented. When functional needs are queried, individuals may report subjective complaints similar to those of individuals in need of hearing instruments; that is, saying that others are constantly mumbling during conversations, having the ability to hear and not fully understand what others are saying, having to turn up the volume on the television or radio to the point at which other family members complain, or reporting that excessive noise in the environment limits the amount of speech understanding. However, these individuals may be adamantly opposed to hearing aid use as an option, which is why assistive technology serves as a feasible alternative.

Subsequent to the functional assessment, it is important to determine the number of environments in which the user will need the assistive technology. Within this realm, a determination of the actual tasks the person will have to perform in terms of job function, activities of daily living, leisure activities, or otherwise is crucial. For instance, using the assistive technology may require the individual to implement modifications in his or her lifestyle for academic or employment purposes. Use of an FM amplification system is often considered as a component of habilitation or rehabilitation to promote academic success in a child with hearing impairment, and written recommendations in an individualized education plan are often made on the type of amplification system a child should use (i.e., a personal or sound-field amplification system). Once this occurs, the chosen amplification system is usually purchased either by the school or the district in which the school resides (K. Takekawa, personal communication, 2003).

After the number of environments in which the user will need the assistive technology is determined, the clinician provides the appropriate technology to match the person's circumstance. Central to the success in use of the assistive technology is choosing one that is not likely to break down, is relatively easy to use, and is durable for an extended period. A complex technology may be more prone to being abandoned, especially if it is selected for someone with cognitive impairments. This person may require an extended period to learn the full capabilities of the technology, or the technology may have extremely delicate parts that can be easily damaged. Finally, an important aspect to consider throughout this entire process is the role of significant others. Significant others in this case refers to parents, spouse, children, or caregiver, because they all play a important role in decision making and ensuring daily use. When in doubt, it may be a good idea to schedule consultations with an audiologist, vision specialist, or other knowledgeable health care providers before any type of assistive technology is obtained.

TRENDS IN AMPLIFICATION AND ASSISTIVE TECHNOLOGY

Current habilitation or rehabilitation for persons who are hard of hearing or deaf can take the form of corrective surgery or provision of amplification, assistive technology, or specialized support services such as interpreters or notetakers. Technology in the twenty-first century for individuals with sensory disability has advanced from low-end paper and pencil communication boards and large bulky hardwire devices to more sophisticated computers and wireless technology (Rothstein & Everson, 1995). Regardless of hearing status, most individuals with (or without) hearing impairment are not innately versed in the mechanics or the communication strategies needed for successful use of amplification and assistive technology. One of the biggest problems facing successful system use is lack of support as well as lack of knowledge of the numerous options available for improving communication. Many in the general public assume that once the amplification or assistive technology is provided, there is no longer a problem. This gap between the lack of understanding and effective use of the equipment is the rationale behind the (re)habilitative patient management principles of many orientation programs.

Quality of life improvement in terms of reducing a hearing handicap and improving physical and mental health functioning are well-established components of the rehabilitation process (Keith, 1994). Most habilitation or rehabilitation programs work to change the perception of what constitutes a hearing handicap and to improve a person's physical and mental health functioning by furnishing educational materials on hearing loss, support counseling, amplification, and assistive technology; setting realistic expectations to assist in better communication; and developing assertive listening strategies to improve communication (Abrahamson, 1991; Abrams, Hnath-Chisolm, Guerreiro, & Ritterman, 1992; Kricos, 1997; Lesner, 2003). This type of orientation process usually involves first-time users of amplification, and the overall success of using (re)habilitative efforts to maximize benefit is closely related to the extent of the program. This premise is based on the fact that programs vary from individualized hearing aid and assistive technology instruction to well-organized group environments that focus not only on the person with the hearing loss but also on their spouses and significant other(s). Resources that provide information about how amplification and assistive technology enable persons with disabilities to experience full participation in activities of daily living are also available via the World Wide Web (www.loc.gov/nls) (National Library Service for the Blind and Physically Handicapped, 2000).

Strategies that enhance communication include optimizing the environment and the speaker–listener relationship. To optimize the environment, there should be good signal-to-noise ratios, increased lighting, and decreased reverberation through the use of drapes and carpeting, because ambient noise can interfere with understanding of speech (Crandell et al., 1995). Similarly, to optimize the speaker–listener relationship, speakers should keep their mouths highly visible; provide concise, highly redundant messages; speak slowly and clearly; indicate changes in topic; and be sensitive to the fatigue level of the listener. Finally, all listeners should be self-advocates for improving communication, such as asking for their communication partner(s) to repeat missed pieces of the conversation and requesting clarifications as necessary.

CONCLUSIONS

Despite improvements in technology and health care, the number of individuals with disabilities and the complexity of needs they and their families experience continues to increase. In response to these needs, specialized technology has been developed to help people with disabilities become more independent and more involved in the activities in their homes, schools, and communities (Berry and Ignash, 2003). The usefulness of amplification and assistive technology for individuals with hearing impairment depends greatly on the type of communication needed and on the amount of residual hearing ability. The service system for people with disabilities has changed from an institutional-based medical model to a more collaborative habilitation or rehabilitation model, and more attention should be given to developing and supporting the providers involved. For instance, even a mild hearing loss in a child can sabotage the development of academic competencies, and there is a growing population of school children with mild to moderate hearing loss (Hawkins, 1984; Hick and Tharpe, 2002). Unfortunately, there are far too few audiologists employed in educational settings (approximately 700 nationally), with an average ratio of 1 audiologist for every 12,000 children, but some audiologists have 100,000 children or more to manage (Flexer, 1990; K. Takekawa, personal communication, 2003; Wilson-Vlotman & Blair, 1986).

Besides identifying the impact of psychosocial, economic, and physical factors on the patient's perceived handicap, the clinician must also consider how these factors influence the best choice of hearing aid styles and assistive technologies for the patient. Economic factors will always play a pivotal role in determining whether the client will be able to afford certain hearing instruments or assistive technology. Psychosocial factors such as the patient's family support and personal self-concept can also affect whether patients choose to use more sophisticated hearing instrument circuitry options. Failure to provide adequate medical and other services for people with disabilities can jeopardize their safety and health, and a good working relationship with the hearing health care professional is a necessary component in this process.

ACKNOWLEDGMENTS

The author acknowledges a number of persons who supplied data or information used in the preparation of this chapter: Michele Ahlman, Cynthia Armas, Jill Kanda, Jason Kaufman, Filiesha LeRand, Eva Leung, Judith Mason, Kris Souza, Kristine Takekawa, Laura Voll, Joan Wylie, Jamie Young, and Erin Zakahi. The Web sites provided in the chapter were current at the time the chapter was written. Because of the transitory nature of Web sites, continued availability at the uniform resource locators (URLs) mentioned herein is not guaranteed.

REFERENCES

Abrahamson, J. (1991). Teaching coping strategies: A client education approach to aural rehabilitation. *Journal of the Academy of Rehabilitative Audiology, 24,* 43–53.

Abrams, H., Hnath-Chisolm, T., Guerreiro, S., & Ritterman, S. (1992). The effects of intervention strategy on self-perception of hearing handicap. *Ear and Hearing, 13,* 371–377.

Allen, J., Hall, J., & Jeng, P. (1990). Loudness growth in 1/2-octave bands (LGOB)—A procedure for the assessment of loudness. *Journal of the Acoustical Society of America, 88,* 745–753.

Berger, K. (1984). *The hearing aid—Its operation and development.* Livonia, MI: National Hearing Aid Society.

Berry, B. E., & Ignash, S. (2003). Assistive technology: Providing independence for individuals with disabilities. *Rehabilitation Nursing, 28,* 6–14.

Byrne, D., & Tonisson, W. (1976). Selecting the gain of hearing aids for persons with sensorineural hearing impairments. *Scandinavian Audiology, 5,* 51–59.

Cornelisse, L., Seewald, R., & Jamieson, D. (1995). The input/output formula: A theoretical approach to the fitting of personal amplification devices. *Journal of the Acoustical Society of America, 97,* 1854–1864.

Cox, R. M. (1995). Using loudness data for hearing aid selection: The IHAFF approach. *The Hearing Journal, 48,* 10, 39–44.

Cox, R. M., & Alexander, G. C. (1995). The abbreviated profile of hearing aid benefit. *Ear and Hearing, 16,* 176–186.

Cox, R. M., & Rivera, I. M. (1992). Predictability and reliability of hearing aid benefit measured using the PHAB. *Journal of the American Academy of Audiology, 3,* 242–254.

Crandell, C., Smaldino, J., & Flexer, C. (1995). *Sound field amplification: Theory and practical applications.* San Diego: Singular.

Dalzell, L., Orlando, M., MacDonald, M., Berg, A., Bradley, M., Cacace, A., et al. (2000). The New York State universal newborn hearing screening demonstration project: Ages of hearing loss identification, hearing aid fitting, and enrollment in early intervention. *Ear and Hearing, 21,* 118–130.

Dillon, H. (1999). NAL-NL-1: A new prescriptive fitting procedure for non-linear hearing aids. *The Hearing Journal, 52,* 10–16.

Dillon, H. (2001). *Hearing aids.* New York: Thieme.

Flexer, C. (1990). Audiological rehabilitation in the schools. *ASHA, 32,* 44–45.

Flexer, C. (1999). *Facilitating hearing and listening in young children* (2nd ed.). San Diego: Singular.

Franks, J. R., & Beckmann, N. J. (1985). Rejection of hearing aids: Attitudes of a geriatric sample. *Ear and Hearing, 6,* 161–166.

Hawkins, D. B. (1984). Comparisons of speech recognition in noise by mildly-to-moderately hearing-impaired children using hearing aids and FM systems. *Journal of Speech and Hearing Disorders, 49,* 409–418.

Hick, C. B., & Tharpe, A. M. (2002). Listening effort and fatigue in school-age children with and without hearing loss. *Journal of Speech Language and Hearing Research, 45,* 573–584.

Humes, L. E., Halling, D., & Coughlin, M. (1996). Reliability and stability of various hearing-aid outcome measures in a group of elderly hearing-aid wearers. *Journal of Speech and Hearing Research, 39,* 923–935.

Keith, R. A. (1994). Functional status and health status. *Archives of Physical Medicine and Rehabilitation, 75,* 478–483.

Killion, M. C., & Fikret-Pasa, S. (1993). The 3 types of sensorineural hearing loss: Loudness and intelligibility considerations. *The Hearing Journal, 46,* 31–36.

Kochkin, S. (1992). MarkeTrak III identifies key factors in determining consumer satisfaction. *The Hearing Journal, 45,* 39–44.

Kochkin, S. (1993). MarkeTrak III: Why 20 million in US don't use hearing aids for their hearing loss. *The Hearing Journal, 46,* 20–27.

Kochkin, S. (1998). MarkeTrak IV: Correlates of hearing aid purchase intent. *The Hearing Journal, 51,* 30–41.

Kricos, P. B. (1997). Audiologic rehabilitation for the elderly: A collaborative approach. *The Hearing Journal, 50,* 10–19.

Lesner, S. A. (2003). Candidacy and management of assistive listening devices: Special needs of the elderly. *International Journal of Audiology, 42*(Suppl. 2), S68–S76.

Lin, H. C., Shu, M. T., Chang, K. C., & Bruna, S. M. (2002). A universal newborn hearing screening program in Taiwan. *International Journal of Pediatric Otorhinolaryngology, 63,* 209–218.

Lucks-Mendel, L., Danhauer, J. L., & Singh, S. (1999). *Singular's illustrated dictionary of audiology.* San Diego: Singular.

Lybarger, S. F. (1988). A historical overview. In R. E. Sandlin (Ed.). *Handbook of hearing aid amplification*, (Vol. I, pp. 1–29). Boston: College Hill Press.

Mark, P. (2000). The swing generation: Challenges and opportunities in the new millennium. *The Hearing Review, 7*, 24–28.

Mason, J. A., & Herrmann, K. R. (1998). Universal infant hearing screening by automated auditory brainstem response measurement. *Pediatrics, 101*, 221–228.

McCandless, G. A., & Lyregaard, P. E. (1983). Prescription of gain/output (POGO) for hearing aids. *Hearing Instruments, 34*, 16–21.

McCarthy, P. (1997). Value of self-assessment scales in measuring hearing aid benefit. *Seminars in Hearing, 18*, 13–17.

Molnar, B., Gergely, J., Toth, G., Pronai, L., Zagoni, T., Papik, K., et al. (2000). Development of a speech-based dialogue system for report dictation and machine control in the endoscopic laboratory. *Endoscopy, 32*, 58–61.

Mueller, H. G., Hawkins, D. B., & Northern, J. L. (1992). *Probe microphone measurements: Hearing aid selection and assessment.* San Diego: Singular.

National Library Service for the Blind and Physically Handicapped (2000). *Assistive technology: A selective bibliography.* Number 00-01. Washington, DC: The Library of Congress.

Newman, C. W., Weinstein, B. E., Jacobson, G. P., & Hug, G. A. (1990). The Hearing Handicap Inventory for Adults: Psychometric adequacy and audiometric correlates. *Ear and Hearing, 11*, 430–433.

Rothstein, R., & Everson, J. M. (1995). Assistive technology for individuals with sensory impairments. In K. F. Flippo, K. J. Inge, & J. M. Barcus (Eds.). *Assistive technology: A resource for school, work, and community* (pp. 105–132). Baltimore: Paul H. Brookes.

Sakai, Y., Watanabe, T., & Kaga, K. (2002). Auditory brainstem responses and usefulness of hearing aids in hearing impaired children with Cornelia de Lange syndrome. *International Journal of Pediatric Otorhinolaryngology, 66*, 63–69.

Sutton, J. (1997). Speech-to-text: the next revelation for recording data. *Radiology Management, 19*, 50–53.

Technology-Related Assistance for Individuals with Disabilities Act of 1988, P.L. 100–407 (1988, August 19). Title 29, U.S.C. 2201 *et seq. U.S. Statutes at Large, 102*, 1044–1065.

Valente, M. (Ed.). (2002a). *Hearing aids: Standards, options, and limitations* (2nd ed.). New York: Thieme.

Valente, M. (Ed.). (2002b). *Strategies for selecting and verifying hearing aid fittings* (2nd ed.). New York: Thieme.

Valente, M., & VanVliet, D. (1997). The independent hearing aid fitting forum (IHAFF) protocol. *Trends in Amplification, 2*, 6–35.

Ventry, I. M., & Weinstein, B. E. (1982). The hearing handicap inventory for the elderly: A new tool. *Ear and Hearing, 3*, 128–134.

Vonlanthen, A. (2000). *Hearing instrument technology for the hearing healthcare professional* (2nd ed.). San Diego: Singular.

Wilson-Vlotman, A. L., & Blair, J. C. (1986). A survey of audiologists working full-time in school systems. *ASHA, 28*, 33–38.

Augmentative and Alternative Communication

Mary Jean J. Dyczko, M.A., CCC/SLP, TSHH, ATP
NYS Licensed Speech-Language Pathologist
RESNA Certified Assistive Technology Practitioner
Practicing Augmentative and Alternative Communication Specialist
New York, NY

Nancy Lenhart Jones, M.S., CCC/SLP, TSHH, ATP
NYS Licensed Speech-Language Pathologist
RESNA Certified Assistive Technology Practitioner
Practicing Augmentative and Alternative Communication Specialist
New York, NY

Aural Rehabilitation for People with Disabilities
Copyright © 2005, Elsevier Inc. All rights reserved.

Training
Summary
References
Selected Readings

Communication is the transmission of one's thoughts, ideas, and wants to another individual or group of individuals. Communication is typically expressed using speech, facial expressions, body language, gestures, and written letters or e-mails. Some individuals have difficulties expressing their wants and needs through traditional means (i.e., speech), and they require assistance for expressing themselves. Various disabilities can affect an individual's ability to speak or write. Augmentative and alternative communication (AAC) systems are methods that are used to help individuals communicate more effectively. Therefore the goal of AAC is effective, quick, and accurate communication.

WHAT IS AUGMENTATIVE AND ALTERNATIVE COMMUNICATION?

"Individuals with severe communication disorders are those who may benefit from [AAC]—those for whom gestural, speech and/or written communication is temporarily or permanently inadequate to meet all of their communication needs. . . . Although some of these individuals may be able to produce a limited amount of speech, it is inadequate to meet their varied communication needs" (American Speech-Language Hearing Association [ASHA], 1989, pp. 107–110). "Augmentative and Alternative Communication is an area of clinical practice that attempts to compensate (either temporarily or permanently) for the impairment and disability patterns of individuals with severe expressive communication disorders (i.e., the severely speech-language impaired)" (ASHA, 1991, p. 10). Beukelman, Yorkston, & Dowden (1985) defined augmentative and alternative communication ". . . as any approach designed to support, enhance, or augment the communication of individuals who are not independent verbal communicators in all situations" (p. 3). Augmentative communication is something used in addition to one's speech, whereas alternative communication is used in place of one's speech.

Individuals with various disabilities can be assisted by AAC techniques. Regardless of disability, age, or background, AAC users have one thing in common: they are unable to effectively communicate everything that they want using their current modes of communication. Typically, an individual's communication is expressed via speech, facial expressions, gestures, and writing. Many disabilities may impair one or all of these modes of communication. A disability may occur at any time in a person's life. Congenital or developmental disabilities, which occur before, at, or around the time of birth, may include disorders such as cerebral palsy, developmental delays, mental retardation, Down's syndrome, hearing impairment, and autism. Acquired disorders are impairments that are sustained after birth, such as hearing impairment and mutism, and can be caused by events such as traumatic brain injury, cerebrovascular accidents (e.g., stroke), spinal cord injury, mutism, hearing impairment, and laryngectomy. A progressive disability is identified when an individual's abilities decline or degenerate over time; examples include multiple sclerosis, amyotrophic lateral sclerosis (Lou Gehrig's disease), and Parkinson's disease.

These disabilities can affect one's ability to communicate in varying degrees. Some individuals will experience minor difficulties expressing themselves and may only need AAC to repair breakdowns in communication. Another group of individuals may be left with unintelligible speech (i.e., speech that is not easily understood by a communication partner); for these individuals AAC has a larger role in their total communication interactions. Others may be unable to speak or write and will depend on AAC as their primary mode of communication. Some individuals may experience a temporary loss in their ability to speak. These include people with a tracheostomy, those who have had long-term intubation, those who have experienced a mental or physical trauma, and those who have had long-term or chronic laryngitis. These individuals may require short-term or temporary use of AAC techniques.

Individuals who present with minor difficulties expressing themselves, specifically related to low-volume and mild speech intelligibility issues, may benefit from the use of amplification systems and speech processors. Amplification systems and speech processors are designed to enhance an individual's current verbal output. Amplification systems increase speech volume, whereas speech processors not only increase volume but also clarify speech.

Those individuals who exhibit more difficulties expressing themselves verbally may require alternative forms of communication in addition to their speech, specifically AAC.

Since its inception, the philosophy of AAC and its use in clinical practice have changed dramatically. Research and knowledge of individuals with disabilities has increased, and this increase has helped to facilitate developments in the field of AAC. Various laws have been enacted and legislative decisions have been made to ensure that individuals with disabilities receive the services (i.e., AAC evaluation and training) that they need to facilitate independence. Legislative decisions include, but are not limited to, the Rehabilitation Act of 1973 (P.L. 93-112), the Consolidated Omnibus Budget Reconciliation Act of 1986 (P.L. 99-509), the Technology-Related Assistance for Individuals with Disabilities Act of 1988 (Tech Act) (P.L. 100-407) and its amendment in 1994 (P.L. 103-218), the Americans with Disabilities Act (ADA) of 1990 (P.L. 101-336), and the Individuals with Disabilities Education Act (IDEA) (P.L. 101-476) (Cook and Hussey, 1995). All these legislative decisions, in addition to others, facilitate independence and educational, medical, and employment support for individuals with disabilities.

Over the years, many changes within the field of AAC have been seen (e.g., the acceptance of AAC in communities, the types and number of available communication systems, the type of vocabulary used in AAC systems, and the number of funding agencies). AAC is a growing field in which new communication devices and access methods are constantly being introduced. Technologic advancements have enabled electronic communication systems to become smaller and include various advanced features. Continual growth in the field of AAC provides individuals with a larger selection of communication systems to find the one that most optimally meets their needs.

AAC is used to improve language skills. Language skills can be broken down into three segments: receptive, expressive, and pragmatic. Receptive language is the comprehension of language (i.e., commands and language concepts [e.g., big versus small]). Expressive language is the speech sounds and grammatical rules of language. Pragmatic language is the use of language (i.e., what our message is accomplishing, [e.g., a greeting]).

AAC symbols may be used in various ways to facilitate the learning of language concepts and understanding of the spoken word. Visual cues—the pairing of an AAC photograph or symbol with the verbal word—enhance the learning of a specific word, concept, or command. Therefore vocabulary growth and reading can be aided by the use of AAC. Transition boards or schedules use AAC photographs and symbols as visual representations of the events or activities in one's day. This enables an individual to anticipate what will happen in his or her day on a more concrete level.

The goal of AAC is communication. Using AAC, an individual can gain attention; make choices; request; protest; comment; greet; ask and answer questions; request clarification; gain information; and regulate a conversation, activity, or his or her environment. These pragmatic functions can be expressed using simple, concrete AAC systems or more abstract, complex systems.

WHAT AFFECTS THE TYPE OF AN AUGMENTATIVE AND ALTERNATIVE COMMUNICATION SYSTEM?

Language and cognitive skills and visual, auditory, and motor/positioning status play an important role in the design and use of AAC systems.

RECEPTIVE LANGUAGE SKILLS AND COGNITION

Cognitive and receptive language skills of the individual determine the complexity of the AAC system. Basic cognitive and receptive language skills are needed to use the simplest forms of AAC. They include object permanence, cause and effect skills, the following of one-step commands, comprehension of simple language concepts, eye contact or awareness of objects, identification of objects, motivation to communicate, and communicative intent (purposeful communication). More complex AAC systems require advanced receptive language and cognitive skills. These skills include: the following of multistep commands; the identification of photographs, picture symbols, letters, or the written word; literacy skills; sequencing skills; and the comprehension of more abstract language concepts. If an individual does not exhibit the skills needed for a basic AAC system, then he or she should be trained in the necessary prerequisite skills. When an individual has these skills and is using a basic AAC system, training should continue to develop the skills necessary for a more advanced AAC system that provides access to more vocabulary. Receptive language skills help to determine which symbols are most appropriate for the AAC system.

Symbol Set

The vocabulary items within an AAC system are called a *symbol set*. Vocabulary items vary in content and complexity. The symbol set can contain vocabulary items that range from very concrete (i.e., use of objects) to abstract (i.e., use of words). Developmentally, language is learned through objects first and then through more abstract representations; such as photographs, line drawings or symbols, and words (Table 9.1) Letter boards (communication boards that resemble keyboards) and word boards represent the most abstract symbol set. An individual's development within the symbol set hierarchy will determine the symbol set used on his or her communication system. The specific symbol set comprises one symbol type (i.e., objects) or a combination of symbol types (i.e., objects and photographs or photographs and picture symbols). When a symbol set contains multiple symbol types, the set can then be called a flexible symbol set.

Many commercial picture symbol libraries are available, including Picture Communication Symbols (Mayer-Johnson, Inc., Solana Beach, CA), DynaSyms (DynaVox Systems LLC, a division of Sunrise Medical, Inc., Pittsburgh, PA), and Minspeak[7] (Baker, 1982) to name a few. These libraries vary in the level of symbol abstractness. Some symbol sets contain symbols that depict only one vocabulary item per symbol (i.e., a picture symbol of an apple expresses "apple"). Other symbol sets contain symbols that have multiple meanings (i.e., picture symbol of an apple can represent the words "apple," "fruit," or "eat") depending on its combination with other symbols (called *semantic compaction* [e.g., Unity]) (Badman et al., 1995). The library chosen should reflect the user's cognitive

Table 9.1

Hierarchy of Symbol Set (from Most Concrete to Most Abstract)

Object level
- Exact object
- Partial object (e.g., label on bottle of bubble solution to represent bubbles)
- Associated object (e.g., spoon to represent lunchtime)
- Miniature object

Photographic level
- Color photograph of exact object with no background
- Black and white photograph of exact object with no background
- Color photograph with background
- Black and white photograph with background

Picture symbol level
- Color line drawing or picture symbol
- Black and white line drawing or picture symbol

Word level
- Whole word, phrase, or sentence
- Spelling

developmental level. Symbol sets can include one symbol library or a combination of two or more libraries.

A picture symbol may be used to represent a single word, phrase, sentence, or extended paragraph. When symbols represent single words or phrases, they may be combined or strung together to construct novel sentences (i.e., "I" + "want" + "to go" + "home" produces the grammatically correct sentence "I want to go home."). Communication systems can also contain single letters, words, phrases, or sentences. Letters can be used to spell words to construct novel utterances.

Morse code (Vanderheiden & Lloyd, 1986) is an international system that uses dashes and dots to spell out words and sentences. The dashes and dots are combined in a predetermined way to produce letters of the alphabet, punctuation, and numbers. Braille (Scholl, 1986) is a tactile symbol system that uses six embossed dots to represent letters of the alphabet, parts of words, and entire words. The way that the dots are arranged determines their meaning. Braille is typically used by individuals who are visually impaired or dual sensory impaired. Both Morse code and Braille can be used on communication systems.

AAC symbols or photographs, Braille, and Morse code may be used in various ways to facilitate the learning of language concepts and understanding of the spoken word. Visual cues with the verbal word enhances the learning of a specific word, concept, or command. In this way, vocabulary growth and reading can be aided by the use of AAC. Transition boards or schedules may use AAC photographs or symbols, Braille, Morse code, or words as visual representations of the events or activities in one's day. This enables an individual to anticipate what will happen in his or her day in a more concrete way than with spoken words alone.

In a communication system, the number of cells (that may contain symbols, words, or letters) with the spaces between them is called the *symbol grid*. The amount of symbols placed on a communication system depends on the grid size. Within a specific area, as the number of symbols increase, the size of those symbols decreases (i.e., given a 3 inch by 3 inch symbol grid one can have one 3 inch by 3 inch symbol or nine 1 inch by 1 inch symbols). In some communication systems the size of the symbol grid is limited (only a few grids are available for that system), and others allow for varied symbol grids (multiple numbers of possible grids are available) or adjustable symbol grids (can create any number of grid designs).

VISION SKILLS

An individual's visual skills (visual fixation, tracking, acuity, and perceptual skills) will determine how his or her communication system will look. Visual skills determine symbol size, the number of symbols used, the symbol grid, and symbol set placement. Although some people can identify an individual 1 inch by 1 inch symbol, they may have difficulty discriminating that symbol when it is surrounded by 20 other symbols. This visual overstimulation can easily be rectified by either decreasing the total number of symbols on the grid or by increasing the size of the symbols.

It is important to be aware of any and all visual deficits an individual has. If an individual has a left field cut, all visual stimuli should be presented on his or her right side. When an individual is blind or legally blind or has impaired vision, tactile symbol sets (i.e., symbols that use texture) or auditory prompts (i.e., the label of the vocabulary item is spoken before selection) can be used to aid in symbol recognition. The use of colors may also aid visual recognition (e.g., the use of black symbols on a yellow background). If an individual has visual processing difficulties, these difficulties need to be identified to make the appropriate accommodations to his or her AAC system. Some AAC users with visual processing difficulties may benefit from the use of auditory prompts because they cue the user as to what the vocabulary items are.

AUDITORY SKILLS

An individual's auditory skills (i.e., auditory acuity and processing) are important in the design of and training to use an AAC system. These skills will determine how information is presented (i.e., whether auditory or visual input is used and to what degree). If an individual has a hearing impairment, perhaps an increase in volume is all that is needed to facilitate comprehension of the vocabulary items. If an individual has no functional hearing, then sign language or visual cues will be needed to aid in the learning of his or her communication system. Hypersensitivity and auditory processing difficulties need to be identified and addressed when one designs and trains an individual to use an AAC system.

Electronic AAC systems use various voice output types. It is important to make sure that the AAC user can hear and comprehend the speech produced by his or her communication system. If an individual has a hearing impairment, the external speakers may be needed to aid in the comprehension of his or her selection. If the user has no functional hearing, then the AAC system may need to have visual output (i.e., a typed message) or tactile feedback so the user knows he or she has made a selection. When one works with an individual who has a hearing loss or is deaf in one ear, it is important to make sure that the speaker of the communication system is near his or her good ear.

PHYSICAL/MOTOR ISSUES

An individual's physical status and motor skills play an important role in the type and design of an AAC system. Whether an individual is ambulatory or uses a wheelchair will affect the size and weight of the communication system. An ambulatory individual will need a lightweight and portable system to allow him or her to carry and use the AAC system in all environments. Because communication systems can be physically attached to wheelchairs, walkers, strollers, or canes, the weight and portability of the system is less of an issue if the individual is not ambulatory.

Seating and positioning are imperative because all mobility comes from a stable base. The reason it is easier to eat when sitting as opposed to standing or standing on one foot is because one has a more stable base when sitting. A stable base can usually be achieved by 90-degree angles at the hips and knees. This base will allow for more neutral muscle tone and will facilitate optimal range of movement in all limbs, the trunk, and the head. To achieve a stable base, individuals with varying degrees of muscle tone will have different positioning needs. When an individual demonstrates hyperextension patterns, it may be beneficial to place him or her in flexion (i.e., less than 90-degree angle). If an individual presents with a limited range of motion, then a smaller communication system would be necessary to accommodate his or her range. An individual with a larger range of motion would be able to access items on a larger communication system.

A controlled, volitional, and reliable movement of a body part is essential for accessing vocabulary items on a communication system. The movement can be as typical as a finger touch or as atypical as an eye blink. This movement must be able to be performed with accuracy, relative ease, and the least amount of fatigue as possible. This will ensure that vocabulary selections will be done in a timely manner and that the individual will be able to communicate throughout his or her day.

Access Techniques

There are two ways to access a communication system. These access techniques are direct selection and indirect selection or scanning.

Direct Selection

Direct selection is an independent, one-to-one correspondence between a person's body and the communication system. A body part can physically touch the system or can hold something that touches vocabulary items on the communication system. Some of the ways the individual can directly access a vocabulary item are by using a finger, thumb, fist, open hand, elbow, foot, toe, or chin. The individual can also use a pointer that is attached to or held by a finger, hand, mouth, or head to directly select items on a communication system. Keyguards may be used to facilitate an increase in accurate accessing when a body part or pointer is used by isolating vocabulary items on the communication system. Use of a keyguard is warranted when an individual demonstrates difficulty accessing one vocabulary item at a time. Keyguards are typically made of plastic, which contains cut-out shapes that conform to the symbols on the AAC system. They are commercially available, can be made to order from certain manufacturers, or can be made by support staff. Direct selection can also be achieved by the use of indicators. Indicators are light pointers, laser pointers, infrared beams, and optical indicators. An emulated mouse (i.e., any device that substitutes for and performs the actions of a standard mouse) or joystick can also be used to directly select items on a communication device. Adaptations can be made to joysticks to accommodate for limited physical abilities (i.e., enlarging the diameter of the joystick to facilitate better control for an individual who presents with a loose grasp).

Indirect Selection or Scanning

Indirect selection or scanning is a dependent, nondirect way of accessing items on a communication system. Vocabulary items are presented to the AAC user, and a selection is made when he or she makes a predetermined response or movement. Any nonelectronic communication system may be manually scanned; for example, the communication partner points to and says each item and the AAC user indicates a selection using a head nod.

Many electronic communication devices contain scanning as a selection technique. As the vocabulary items are being scanned they may be visually highlighted (e.g., with lights or color) or auditorally highlighted (e.g., with beeps or verbal cues). The AAC user makes his or her selection by accessing a switch, which in turn activates the communication device. We use switches in our everyday lives; for example, when we push a light switch it activates or turns on the light. There are various switches that can be accessed by many different body parts. A controlled volitional movement of a body part is needed to access a switch. The identified body part is called the switch site. The movement of that body part is what is going to activate the switch. Once the switch site and body part movement have been identified, then a switch can be matched to them. Switches come in all sizes, shapes, and colors to accommodate different switch sites. Switches can be activated by various methods, for example, touch, release, breath, squeeze, and tilt or movement of the switch. Switches also accommodate different degrees of pressure (e.g., a foot stomp or a slight finger touch). In reality, once a reliable switch site and body part movement have been identified, a switch can be found or adapted for it.

Vocabulary items can be scanned in many different patterns. Linear scanning is the scanning of each item consecutively from left to right. Circular scanning is clockwise scanning of items. Row and column scanning is consecutive scanning of rows from top to bottom and, once a row is selected, scanning of each column within that row from left to right. Column and row scanning is consecutive scanning of columns from left to right and, once a column is selected, scanning of each row within that column from top to bottom. Quadrant scanning is clockwise scanning of the entire display in four quadrants, and, once a quadrant is selected, scanning of items row by row and then column by column. Top and bottom scanning is scanning of the top and bottom halves of the display and then scanning of items row by row and column by column. Left and right scanning is scanning of the left and right halves of the display and then scanning of items row by row and column by column. Left, center, or right scanning is scanning of the left, center, and right quadrants of the display first and then scanning of items row by row and column by column. Group scanning is scanning of set groups in the display first and then scanning of items row by row and column by column. The scanning pattern chosen is determined by skill of the individual AAC user and by speed of communication. The amount of time in between vocabulary choices is called *scan timing*. Scan timing provides the AAC user with enough time to activate his or her switch. Scan timing is adjusted to accommodate the skills of the AAC user to produce accurate selection of targeted vocabulary items.

Various scan types are available in electronic communication devices. With auto scan the vocabulary items are automatically scanned in a preset time-dependent pattern until the AAC user activates his or her switch to make a selection. Inverse scanning is used when an AAC user can better release a switch, then activate it. Scanning begins in a preset time-dependent pattern when the AAC user activates his or her switch and a selection is made upon release of the switch. Step scan is not time dependent. The step scan is controlled by the AAC user, not by the passage of time. The user scans vocabulary items along a preset pattern with each activation of his or her switch. A selection is made when the user either stops hitting the switch for a predetermined period or hits a second switch.

Auditory scanning of vocabulary items is an option on some electronic devices. It provides the individual with verbal prompts or cues (i.e., label) and the visual scanning of vocabulary items. Auditory scanning provides the AAC user with additional feedback to help cue him or her to the choices that are being scanned. It can be used to facilitate training for scanning, as extra cues for users who are cognitively impaired, for those who are more auditory learners than visual learners, and for those who are visually impaired.

AUGMENTATIVE AND ALTERNATIVE COMMUNICATION SYSTEMS

A variety of AAC systems are currently available. All systems are set up to work toward a common goal: to improve expressive language skills and functional communication. There are two basic types of AAC systems: manual communication systems and electronic communication systems. Usually individuals have both manual and electronic systems, which are used at different times and in different environments. Both manual and electronic communication systems have various symbol types as well as symbol grids. The main difference between the types is that one is electronic and one is not. Another difference is in the number of features available. Manual communication systems are typically designed from scratch for a specific individual and his or her communication, physical, and sensory (i.e., visual and hearing) needs. Electronic communication systems are manufactured with a number of features. It is then up to the AAC user's support staff (i.e., the speech–language pathologist and assistive technology practitioner) to customize the system to meet his or her communication, physical, and sensory needs. The simplicity or complexity of a user's communication system, whether it is manual or electronic, depends on his or her cognitive, receptive language, visual, and physical skills and expressive needs (i.e., amount of vocabulary needed).

Both electronic and manual communication systems may use similar vocabulary retrieval methods. A single vocabulary selection can produce a single letter (e.g., "w"), a word (e.g., "want"), a phrase, (e.g. "I want to go"), a sentence (e.g., "I want to go to the park"), or a whole paragraph (e.g., the Pledge of Allegiance). Vocabulary items can be represented by individual objects, photographs, picture symbols, phrases, single words, or letters.

To ensure that an individual has the vocabulary needed to meet all of his or her communicative needs in all environments, a vocabulary analysis should be conducted. This entails getting vocabulary items from family members, therapists, teachers, employers, and other significant people in the individual's life across all environments. Information may be retrieved through the use of phone calls, lists, prewritten forms, or e-mails. In order to provide the individual with the necessary vocabulary to communicate in all environments it is essential to get information from all potential communication partners. This includes communication interactions that may take place daily (e.g., hello routines) or once a year (e.g., wishing someone happy holidays).

Vocabulary items can be organized in different ways on a communication system. Individual-centered communication boards or displays are designed with specific vocabulary to meet the needs of a particular AAC user (e.g., a sportscaster would have vocabulary words to talk about sports, whereas a chef needs an extensive food vocabulary). They also contain commonly used words and phrases (e.g., husband's name and "I need help"). These boards or displays are composed of the AAC user's primary and most important vocabulary items. Other boards or displays are constructed with vocabulary words that are specific to an activity regardless of the individual user (e.g., bubbles or an art project); these are called *activity-centered boards or displays*. Other boards or displays are category based (e.g., food or clothing). Category and activity-centered boards are composed of secondary vocabulary items for the AAC user. These vocabulary items are environment specific and may not be used daily. Some communication systems include both individual- and activity-centered communication boards or displays.

Individual and activity-centered displays may be organized in various ways. One way to enhance retrieval of vocabulary items is by color coding according to parts of speech. This enables the AAC user to quickly locate items based on grammar and colors. For example, if nouns are yellow and verbs are pink, an AAC user would look at the symbols with a yellow background to find "hamburger." Vocabulary items can be set up within a display so that all parts of speech are together and in order, from left to right, to formulate a grammatically correct sentence (i.e., vocabulary items representing pronouns, verbs, and nouns would be placed in columns from left to right). Some communication displays are produced so that needed vocabulary items are placed in order from left to right following the script of the communication interaction. For example, a greetings overlay may contain the following vocabulary in this order from left to right: "Hello," "How are you?," "I am fine," "What did you do this weekend?," "I had fun this weekend," "Goodbye," and "See you soon."

Communication displays, whether individual- or activity-centered, may be done in one or more languages (e.g., English words to converse with peers and Polish to converse with family members in Poland who do not understand English). With manual systems, the production of various languages is rather simple and depends only on finding someone who can write in those languages. Using various languages in electronic systems with voice output is more complicated. The electronic device itself must have that language as an included feature, the ability to program in a new language, or the ability to alter how words sound phonetically.

The amount of vocabulary needed in an AAC user's communication system depends on his or her receptive language skills and communication needs. Some individuals may present with speech that is usually understood. He or she may only need a few words on an AAC system that can be used when a breakdown in communication occurs (i.e., the communication partner does not understand the AAC user's speech). Others may exhibit more unintelligible speech and may be rarely understood by listeners. These individuals would have communication systems that incorporate a lot of vocabulary to accommodate his or her needs. Communication should be multimodal; more than one mode can be used for the expression of language. For example, an AAC user may signal yes or no responses by the use of traditional head nods, may request using symbols, and may vocalize to gain attention. When one designs a communication system, a specific vocabulary item should not be repeated unless one or more of the AAC user's partners do not understand it. For example, an AAC user who is literate may have a letter board. Although the user can spell out messages, he or she may need to have symbol representation of vocabulary items to communicate with a nonliterate peer or communication partner.

Vocabulary expansion techniques are ways that vocabulary can be retrieved quickly in both electronic and manual communication systems. Vocabulary expansion techniques are rate enhancement features that speed up the communication rate of the AAC user, which in turn saves time and energy (fewer keystrokes or a decreased number of vocabulary selections needed to produce a message). Included are abbreviation expansion, memory keys and built-in phrases, word completion and word prediction, page linking, levels, and semantic compaction.

Abbreviation expansion, memory keys, files, and built-in phrases are techniques in which a combination of letters or numbers represent a phrase, sentence, or paragraph. For example, "HB" when expanded depicts the message "Hey Babe," the phrase "I want to go to the bathroom" can be condensed into two letters and an expansion key "WB=," and the Pledge of Allegiance may be shortened to the expansion "PA." Abbreviated expansions may also be used for common words or phrases that the user often misspells. With manual systems, once the AAC user produces an abbreviation expansion, his or her partner needs to look at a chart or book that lists and defines all of the user's abbreviation expansions. On electronic systems, once the abbreviation expansion is complete, the entire message is produced. Some electronic devices have another rate enhancement feature called *memory keys* or *files* or *built-in phrases*. These can also store messages of varying length (up to a small report) and are accessed via one or two keystrokes. Abbreviation expansion, memory keys, and files can be programmed by the user. Built-in phrases are typically preprogrammed by the device manufacturer.

Word completion and word prediction are rate-enhancement techniques that are used by literate AAC users. Word completion attempts to predict the word the user is beginning to spell. As a letter is selected, words that start with that letter are presented to the user. For example, as one types the letter "h" the words "home," "hello," and "hat" may be presented. When the individual adds the letter "o" the words "home," "hope," and "honesty" may then be presented. Word prediction also attempts to predict the next word from the AAC user on the basis of grammatical rules. For example, if the user spells the word "they," the words "are" and "will" may be predicted but not the word "is." Word completion and word prediction are based on the frequency of use of a standard vocabulary set (based on the general population) or a custom vocabulary set (user's specific way of using and combining words). Electronic systems usually provide the AAC user with word completion and word prediction choices visually and/or auditorally. With manual systems, the AAC user relies on his or her communication partner to verbally "guess" the partially spelled word or predict the next word.

Page linking is a technique used to expand vocabulary by the use of categories or activities. When an AAC user selects a category, a new communication board or display is presented to the user with vocabulary specific to that category. For example, an individual wanting to eat would select or page link to his or her food page. On that page, the AAC user would have a listing of all favorite foods. With manual systems, the changing of pages or boards may be done manually by the AAC user or by his or her communication partner. With electronic devices, page linking is done automatically. When the AAC user selects the category or activity, the page opens up, and vocabulary choices within that category are displayed to the user.

Levels are another vocabulary expansion technique that provide the user with additional vocabulary items. Some electronic systems have the ability to have more than one communication board or page programmed into it at a time. Each programmed board is a level. The levels may be changed manually by the user or communication partner by physically changing the communication board on the display and turning a knob to change to the desired level that has the corresponding preprogrammed vocabulary in it. Other electronic systems can change to the desired level when a specific selection is made. Then it is up to the user or partner to simply change the communication board. Instead of having to physically change a board, some communication displays are designed to present the user with all levels at one time. For example, a cell may be divided into three sections, each representing vocabulary items from a different level. A user selects and locks himself or herself into a level. All selections will contain vocabulary from that locked-in level until the user changes levels. Manual systems are typically designed using the latter method of presenting multiple levels on one communication board.

Semantic compaction (Unity) (Badman et al., 1995) is another vocabulary enhancement technique. Semantic compaction uses symbols or icons that have multiple meanings, as discussed earlier. Because one symbol or icon represents multiple words or phrases, fewer icons need to be presented to the user to express a larger vocabulary. Therefore the user can quickly scan his or her few icons to produce unlimited vocabulary. Some systems contain specific icon combinations, and others let the AAC user decide which symbols should be combined to represent a specific vocabulary item. A few electronic systems contain semantic compaction. They will produce the desired message once the entire combination of symbols has been completed. Some electronic devices will aid the AAC user by a feature called icon prediction. When a symbol is chosen, only the icons that can be combined with the original chosen icon are highlighted (i.e., by a light or by a change in backlight). Manual systems require that the communication partner or listener and the AAC user learn semantic compaction. It is up to the listener to *read and expand* the semantic compaction produced by the AAC user.

A communication device refers to the individual electronic device, whereas a communication system consists of the manual or electronic communication device and its accessories. Accessories to facilitate functional use of the manual system or electronic device may include mounting systems, access method (i.e., pointer, laser, optical indicator, switch, joystick, or mouse emulation), speakers, keyguards, and carry case.

MANUAL COMMUNICATION SYSTEMS

Manual communication systems are nonelectronic forms of AAC that are customized for a particular individual, taking his or her specific skills, vocabulary needs, access issues, and communication needs into account. They can be extremely accommodating with regard to size and shape. Manual communication systems may contain one or a combination of symbol sets (objects, photographs, pictures or symbols, letters, words, and phrases) on the same system. They do not provide voice output and depend on the close proximity of the listener to *read* the AAC user's vocabulary selections. Manual communication systems may be the individual's primary means of communication or may be used as a backup method when his or her electronic device is not available.

Vocabulary items on manual communication systems can be selected directly or indirectly. Direct access consists of pointing with a finger or other body part, the use of a pointer to directly touch a vocabulary item (e.g., a mouth stick that is held in the mouth or a pointer attached to a hand splint), or the use of an indicator (e.g., light or laser pointer). Keyguards may be used to facilitate accurate access of vocabulary items when needed. An indicator can be held or attached to a body part (i.e., on top of the head). The indicator is then placed on or shown on the desired vocabulary item. Manual communication systems can also be accessed indirectly. With manual or partner-assisted scanning, the communication partner or listener scans the vocabulary page for the AAC user (see the earlier section on scanning techniques). The listener verbally or physically cues the AAC user to the vocabulary items, and when the AAC user makes a predetermined response the partner announces the chosen vocabulary item and waits for confirmation.

Manual communication systems consist of communication boards or books or wallets and eyegaze systems. A communication board contains individual displays containing vocabulary items (Fig. 9.1). Communication boards vary greatly in size; they may be as small as an index card or large enough to cover an entire lap tray of a wheelchair. A communication book or wallet is a collection of individual communication boards to provide the AAC user with many vocabulary items. Communication books and wallets are designed to be small, portable, and lightweight. Communication books can be carried or worn with a strap, like a book bag or purse. Communication wallets are smaller than communication books and can be carried in a pocket.

Eyegaze systems can include, but are not limited to, Eye Links (Drinker & Krupoff, 1981) and E-TRANs (Beukelman & Mirenda, 1992). Eyegaze systems use an individual's eyes to point to or select vocabulary targets. Eye Links are clear displays that provide the AAC user with all letters of the alphabet and some words and functions (e.g., end of word, backspace, and finished) (Fig. 9.2). The AAC user points to individual letters to spell out a word or sentence with his or her eyes. The communication listener must move the Eye Link around to attempt to *read* the letters that the AAC user's eye is pointing to. The listener *reads* these letters by moving the Eye Link around until he or she makes direct eye contact with the AAC user. When eye contact is made, the letter in between their eyes is the selected vocabulary item.

E-TRANs (Beukelman & Mirenda, 1992) are constructed of clear Plexiglas or plastic with vocabulary items (i.e., objects, symbols, and words) placed on them (Fig. 9.3). The E-TRAN is usually placed on an AAC user's wheelchair. The AAC user looks at a vocabulary item and his or her partner looks through the opening in the E-TRAN to see what vocabulary item the AAC user is looking at.

The E-TRAN (Beukelman & Mirenda, 1992) differs from the Eye Link (Drinker & Krupoff, 1981) in that it is a more independent, stationary form of communication; the communication partner or listener does not have to physically move the communication display around to read the user's vocabulary selections.

There are many advantages and disadvantages to the use of manual communication systems. Some of them are listed in Table 9.2.

Text continues on page 233

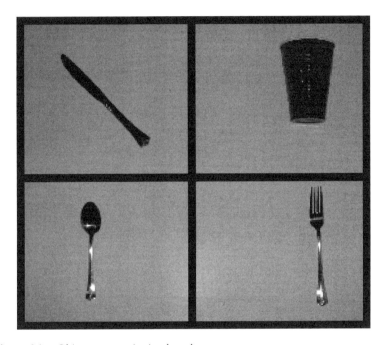

Figure 9.1   Object communication board.

A	B	C	D	E
F	G	H	I	J
K	L	M	N	O
P	Q	R	S	T
U	V	W	X	Y
Z	End of word	Backspace	Mistake	Finished

Figure 9.2   Eye Link board.

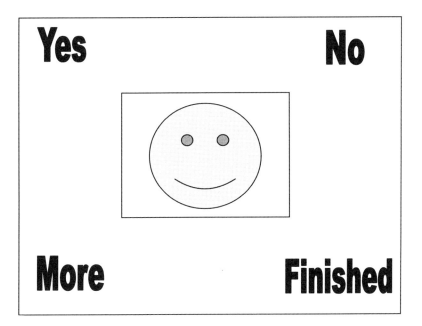

Figure 9.3   Drawing of an E-TRAN.

Table 9.2

Manual Communication Systems

Advantages	Disadvantages
Manual systems can be made portable and lightweight.	Manual systems require more work from the communication partner (e.g., the listener needs to be close by to see all selections).
Manual systems can contain one or a combination of symbol sets (e.g., symbols, photos, or objects).	With a manual system, if the AAC user is a scanner, then communication depends on his or her partner scanning vocabulary selections.
Manual systems can contain vocabulary items in any language.	Because manual systems do not have voice output, they are difficult in group settings.
Manual systems can be created using any size of symbols and symbol grid.	Many people unfortunately do not view the use of manual systems as "communication" because they do not have voice output.
Manual systems can be used in all environments (e.g., pool or bathtub).	Many people unfortunately associate lower cognitive levels with the use of manual systems.
Manual systems are typically more dependable: repairs (e.g., recontacting or regluing) are usually easier and quicker than with electronic systems.	With manual systems, the more vocabulary an AAC user requires, the larger the communication board or the more pages he or she must manually change or flip.
Manual systems typically do not need to be charged or maintained as regularly as electronic systems.	
Manual systems usually require less set up.	
Families of individuals using AAC appear to have less fear of manual systems than of electronic systems.	
Families of individuals using AAC are typically less horrified when a manual system is lost or broken.	

ELECTRONIC COMMUNICATION SYSTEMS

Electronic communication systems require a battery to operate. They come in all sizes and shapes with different features that will assist the AAC user to communicate effectively. Electronic communication devices range from simplistic (single message voice output device) to complex (multimessage or multiaccess device).

As with manual communication systems, vocabulary items on electronic communication devices can be selected directly or indirectly. Direct access consists of pointing with a body part or use of a pointer, indicators, a joystick, or an emulated mouse. Some electronic devices have a touch screen that closely resembles the touch window for computers, automated teller machines, or MetroCard vending machines. With a light touch, the AAC user can access any cell on the screen or display of the communication device. Electronic devices with touch screens have modifications to allow the user ease of access to suit his or her physical status. One modification will allow the user to slide his or her hand across the screen, making no selection until he or she lifts the hand off the desired location or cell on the screen. Keyguards may be needed to improve the accuracy of vocabulary selections. Electronic communication systems can also be accessed indirectly through a switch using scanning (see earlier section on indirect selection or scanning for various scanning options). Some electronic devices have only one means of access (direct selection or scanning), whereas others can be accessed in various ways (i.e., both direct selection and scanning or point, joystick, emulated mouse, and single switch scanning). Electronic devices that can be accessed in two or more ways are said to have multiaccess input methods.

There are many advantages and disadvantages to electronic communication systems. Some of them are listed in Table 9.3. Electronic communication systems have various features that differ among devices to better match the specific needs and skills of the AAC user. Features include, but are not limited to, type of display, output upon vocabulary selection, type of electronic device (dedicated versus nondedicated), availability of environmental control units, and portability. Refer to Table 9.4 for a listing of some electronic communications devices and their specific features.

Text continues on page 272

Table 9.3

Electronic Communication Systems

Advantages	Disadvantages
With the use of electronic systems, the communication partner does not have to assist the user in communication, therefore allowing the AAC user to communicate independently.	With electronic systems, the symbol grid is limited to the size of the display or screen.
The voice output feature that is included in many electronic systems allows independent communication in all environments (e.g., talking on the phone or talking in group settings).	Some electronic systems contain predetermined symbol sizes; therefore, there is little ability to adjust.
Electronic systems usually allow various access methods: direct selection and scanning (multiple access methods are essential for those with progressive disorders).	A limited number of electronic devices allow use of scanned photographs, and when they do, memory becomes an issue.
Some electronic systems have dynamic displays that allow access to a large amount of vocabulary quickly.	Usually the more vocabulary available per page requires either using smaller symbols or using an electronic system with a larger screen, which is often a heavier device that may be portable for the ambulatory user (excludes devices that use semantic encoding).
Some electronic systems contain preprogrammed pages that enable the AAC user to have access to a range of vocabulary quickly.	With electronic systems that contain synthesized voice output, a limited number of languages are available.
Electronic systems that contain digitized voice output allow any language to be programmed.	With electronic systems that contain digitized speech, record time is limited.
Electronic systems that are contained in a computer provide the AAC user with both communication and computer activities (i.e., educational software and Internet access).	Electronic systems require more maintenance (i.e., charging and cost of batteries) and repairs (e.g., more fragile if dropped) that leave the AAC user without a system for a period.
Some electronic systems may contain environmental control units that allow the AAC user to access his or her environment and to communicate.	The use of electronic systems is limited to certain environments (e.g., one would not use it in a pool or bathtub, and some systems with dynamic displays cannot be used in sunlight without a cover).
Some electronic systems may contain auditory prompts that enable or aid visually impaired and cognitively impaired users who scan.	Electronic systems typically require more set-up time.
	Some families have a fear of electronic systems and therefore may not provide the AAC user with the system as often.

Table 9.4

Electronic Communication Devices and Their Features

AAC Device	Voice Output	Display	Vocabulary Size[a]	Vocabulary Expansion	Type of System	Symbol Type	Access Method	Portable/ Light-weight	Symbol Grid[b]	ECU
1-Level-32 Message Communicator Enabling Devices 800-832-8697 www.enablingdevices.com	Digitized	Static	Limited	None	Dedicated	Flexible Symbol Set	Direct Selection	Yes	Limited	No
2 Level Communicator, 2 Level Communicator with Jacks Enabling Devices 800-832-8697 www.enablingdevices.com	Digitized	Static	Limited	Levels	Dedicated	Flexible Symbol Set	Direct Selection	Yes	Limited	No
2/3/6-Level-32 Message Communicator Enabling Devices 800-832-8697 www.enablingdevices.com	Digitized	Static	Medium to Large Depend-ing on Model	Level	Dedicated	Flexible Symbol Set	Direct Selection	Yes	Limited	No

AAC, Augmentive and alternative communication; *ECU,* environmental control unit.

[a]For the purposes of this table, Limited = up to 27 vocabulary items available on communication device, Medium = 28 to 127 vocabulary items available on communication device, Large = 128 or more vocabulary items available on communication device and/or keyboard (which provides an unlimited number of novel vocabulary items).

[b]For the purposes of this table, Limited = 3 or fewer interchangeable symbol grids, Varied = 4 or more interchangeable symbol grids, Adjustable = the ability to create/individualize grids specifically for the AAC user.

(continues)

Table 9.4
(*continued*)

AAC Device	Voice Output	Display	Vocabulary Size	Vocabulary Expansion	Type of System	Symbol Type	Access Method	Portable/ Light-weight	Symbol Grid	ECU
4-Plate Communicator Enabling Devices 800-832-8697 www.enablingdevices.com	Digitized	Static	Limited	None	Dedicated	Flexible Symbol Set	Direct Selection	Yes	Limited	No
4talk4 Penny + Giles Computer Products +44(0)1425-463100 www.penny-gilescp.co.uk	Synthesized	Static	Limited	Levels	Dedicated	Flexible Symbol Set	Direct Selection Switch Access	Yes	Limited	No
6 Level Communicator, 6 Level Communicator with Jacks Enabling Devices 800-832-8697 www.enablingdevices.com	Digitized	Static	Medium	Levels	Dedicated	Flexible Symbol Set	Direct Selection	Yes	Limited	No
7 Level Blue Communication Builder Enabling Devices 800-832-8697 www.enablingdevices.com	Digitized	Static	Large	Level	Dedicated	Flexible Symbol Set	Direct Selection	Yes	Limited	No
AlphaSmart 3000 AlphaSmart Inc. 888-274-0680 www.alphasmart.com	None	Static	Large	Depends on Software Purchased	Nondedicated	Keyboard Text to Speech	Direct Selection	Yes	Varied	No

Device										
AlphaTalker II Prentke Romich Co. 800-262-1933 www.prentrom.com	Digitized	Static	Large	Levels, Unity	Dedicated	Flexible Symbol Set Unity	Multiple Access Methods	Yes	Limited	No
Art[c] ZYGO Industries, Inc. 800-234-6006 www.zygo-usa.com	Synthesized	Color Dynamic	Large	Page Linking	Nondedicated	Flexible Symbol Set	Direct Selection	Yes	Adjustable	No
Auditory Queing Communicator (AQC) Enabling Devices 800-832-8697 www.enablingdevices.com	Digitized	Static	Limited	None	Dedicated	Flexible Symbol Set	Multiple Access Auditory Prompts	Yes	Limited	No
Base Trainer ERI 516-501-0235 www.eridevices.com	Digitized	Static	Limited	None	Dedicated	Flexible Symbol Set	Direct Selection	Yes	Limited	No
Bedside Communicator Enabling Devices 800-832-8697 www.enablingdevices.com	Digitized	Static	Limited	None	Dedicated	Flexible Symbol Set	Scan	No	Limited	No
Big Mac Ablenet 800-322-0956 www.ablenetinc.com	Digitized	Static	Limited	None	Dedicated	Flexible Symbol Set	Direct Selection Switch Access	Yes	Limited	No

[c] A computer only; communication software needs to be ordered with the computer in order for the listed features to be available.

(continues)

238

Table 9.4

(*continued*)

AAC Device	Voice Output	Display	Vocabulary Size	Vocabulary Expansion	Type of System	Symbol Type	Access Method	Portable/ Light-weight	Symbol Grid	ECU
Black Hawk Adam Lab 734-334-1610 www.adamlab.com	Digitized	Static	Medium	Levels	Dedicated	Flexible Symbol Set	Direct Selection	Yes	Limited	No
Box-Talk 16X4, Box-Talk 16X6, Box-Talk 16XL Common Cents 800-805-9278 www.box-talk.com	Digitized	Static	Large	None	Dedicated	Flexible Symbol Set	Multiple Access Methods	Yes	Limited	No
Box-Talk 9 Bi-Level, Box-Talk 16 Bi-Level Common Cents 800-805-9278 www.box-talk.com	Digitized	Static	Limited	Levels	Dedicated	Flexible Symbol Set	Multiple Access Methods	Yes	Limited	No
Box-Talk 9 Auditory, Box-Talk 16 Auditory Common Cents 800-805-9278 www.box-talk.com	Digitized	Static	Limited	None	Dedicated	Flexible Symbol Set	Multiple Access Methods Auditory Scan	Yes	Limited	No

Product										
Box-Talk 9 Standard, Box-Talk 16 Standard Common Cents 800–805–9278 www.box-talk.com	Digitized	Static	Limited	None	Dedicated	Flexible Symbol Set	Multiple Access Methods	Yes	Limited	No
Box-Talk 9 X4, Box-Talk 9X6, Box-Talk 9X8 Common Cents 800–805–9278 www.box-talk.com	Digitized	Static	Medium	None	Dedicated	Flexible Symbol Set	Multiple Access Methods	Yes	Limited	No
Bulletin Board Communicator Enabling Devices 800–832–8697 www.enablingdevices.com	Digitized	Static	Limited	None	Dedicated	Flexible Symbol Set	Scan	No	Limited	No
Cameleon 4 Cambridge Adaptive Communication 12396–461002 www.cameleon-web.com	Synthesized	Color Dynamic	Large	Page Linking Word Prediction Abbreviation Expansion	Nondedicated	Flexible Symbol Set	Multiple Access Methods	No	Adjustable	Yes
Card Communicator Crestwood Communication Aids, Inc. 41-352-5678 www.communicationaids.com	None	Static	Limited	None	Dedicated	Flexible Symbol Set	Scan	No	Limited	No

(continues)

239

Table 9.4

(*continued*)

AAC Device	Voice Output	Display	Vocabulary Size	Vocabulary Expansion	Type of System	Symbol Type	Access Method	Portable/ Light-weight	Symbol Grid	ECU
Carousel Communicator 1 Level 7 Messages Enabling Devices 800-832-8697 www.enablingdevices.com	Digitized	Static	Small	None	Dedicated	Flexible Symbol Type	Direct Selection	No	Limited	No
Carousel Communicator 6 Level 42 Messages Enabling Devices 800-832-8697 www.enablingdevices.com	Digitized	Static	Large	Levels	Dedicated	Flexible Symbol Type	Direct Selection	No	Limited	No
Chat PC Satillo Corp. 330-674-6722 www.saltillo.com	Synthesized Digitized	Color Dynamic	Large	Page Linking	Dedicated	Flexible Symbol Set	Direct Selection	Yes	Varied	No
Chatbox Satillo Corp. 330-674-6722 www.saltillo.com	Digitized	Static	Large	Semantic Encoding Icon Prediction	Dedicated	Unity	Multiple Access Methods	Yes	Varied	No

Product									
Chatbox Dx Satillo Corp. 330–674–6722 www.saltillo.com	Digitized	Static	Large	Semantic Encoding Icon Prediction	Dedicated	Unity	Multiple Access Methods Auditory Scan	Yes	Varied	No
Cheap Talk 4 In–line Scan Enabling Devices 800–832–8697 www.enablingdevices.com	Digitized	Static	Limited	None	Dedicated	Flexible Symbol Set	Scan	Yes	Limited	No
Cheap Talk 4 In–line Series: Direct, Direct and Jacks, Direct and Scan, Direct Scan and Jacks Enabling Devices 800–832–8697 www.enablingdevices.com	Digitized	Static	Limited	None	Dedicated	Flexible Symbol Set	Multiple Access Methods	Yes	Limited	No
Cheap Talk 4 Direct and Jacks with Overlay Option In–line, Cheap Talk 4 Direct and Jacks with Overlay Option Square Enabling Devices 800–832–8697 www.enablingdevices.com	Digitized	Static	Limited	None	Dedicated	Flexible Symbol Set	Direct Selection	Yes	Limited	No

(continues)

Table 9.4

(*continued*)

AAC Device	Voice Output	Display	Vocabulary Size	Vocabulary Expansion	Type of System	Symbol Type	Access Method	Portable/ Light-weight	Symbol Grid	ECU
Cheap Talk 4 Direct with Overlay Option In-line, Cheap Talk 4 Direct with Overlay Option Square Enabling Devices 800–832–8697 www.enablingdevices.com	Digitized	Static	Limited	None	Dedicated	Flexible Symbol Set	Direct Selection	Yes	Limited	No
Cheap Talk 8 Say It Play It Enabling Devices 800–832–8697 www.enablingdevices.com	Digitized	Static	Limited	None	Dedicated	Flexible Symbol Set	Direct Selection	Yes	Limited	No
Cheap Talk 8 Scan Enabling Devices 800–832–8697 www.enablingdevices.com	Digitized	Static	Limited	None	Dedicated	Flexible Symbol Set	Scan	Yes	Limited	No
Cheap Talk 8 Direct and Scan, Cheap Talk 8 Direct and Scan with Jacks Enabling Devices 800–832–8697 www.enablingdevices.com	Digitized	Static	Limited	None	Dedicated	Flexible Symbol Set	Multiple Access Methods	Yes	Limited	No

242

Device / Contact									
Cheap Talk 8 Direct, Cheap Talk 8 Direct and Jacks Enabling Devices 800-832-8697 www.enablingdevices.com	Digitized	Static	Limited	None	Dedicated	Flexible Symbol Set	Direct Selection	Yes	Limited	No
Chipper Adaptivation, Inc. 605-335-4445 www.adaptivation.com	Digitized	Static	Limited	None	Dedicated	Flexible Symbol Set	Direct Selection Switch Access	Yes	Limited	No
Clip Talk Direct Select with Jacks Only, Clip Talk Direct Select and Jacks Enabling Devices 800-832-8697 www.enablingdevices.com	Digitized	None	Limited	None	Dedicated	None	Direct Selection Switch Access with Jacks	Yes	None	No
Communication Builder Enabling Devices 800-832-8697 www.enablingdevices.com	Digitized	Static	Limited	None	Dedicated	Flexible Symbol Set	Direct Selection	Yes	Varied	No
Communicator 25 Gus Communications, Inc. 866-487-1006 www.gusinc.com	Synthesized Digitized	Color Dynamic	Large	Page Linking	Dedicated, Nondedicated (versions)	Flexible Symbol Set	Direct Selection	Yes	Adjustable	No

(continues)

Table 9.4

(*continued*)

AAC Device	Voice Output	Display	Vocabulary Size	Vocabulary Expansion	Type of System	Symbol Type	Access Method	Portable/ Light-weight	Symbol Grid	ECU
Communicator 320 Gus Communications, Inc. 866–487-1006 www.gusinc.com	Synthesized Digitized	Color Dynamic	Large	Page Linking Text to Speech	Dedicated, Nondedicated (versions)	Flexible Symbol Set Keyboard	Direct Selection	Yes	Adjustable	No
Communicator 35 Gus Communications, Inc. 866–487-1006 www.gusinc.com	Synthesized Digitized	Color Dynamic	Large	Page Linking	Dedicated, Nondedicated (versions)	Flexible Symbol Set	Direct Selection	Yes	Adjustable	No
Communicator 3500 Gus Communications, Inc. 866–487-1006 www.gusinc.com	Synthesized Digitized	Color Dynamic	Large	Page Linking	Dedicated, Nondedicated (versions)	Flexible Symbol Set	Direct Selection	Yes	Adjustable	No
Communicator 600 Gus Communications, Inc. 866–487-1006 www.gusinc.com	Synthesized Digitized	Color Dynamic	Large	Page Linking	Dedicated, Nondedicated (versions)	Flexible Symbol Set	Direct Selection	Yes	Adjustable	No
Communiclock Crestwood Communication Aids, Inc. 414-352-5678 www.communicationaids.com	None	Static	Limited	None	Dedicated	Flexible Symbol Set	Scan	Yes	Adjustable	No

Device	Speech	Display	Vocabulary	Levels		Symbol/Input	Access Method	Scan		
Communilight 24 Crestwood Communication Aids, Inc. 414–352–5678 www.communicationaids.com	Digitized	Static	Limited	None	Dedicated	Flexible Symbol Set	Scan	Yes	Limited	No
Crespeaker Crestwood Communication Aids, Inc. 414–352–5678 www.communicationaids.com	Synthesized	Static	Large	Built in Phrases	Nondedicated	Keyboard with Text to Speech	Direct Selection	Yes	Limited	No
Dana AlphaSmart Inc. 888–274–0680 www.alphasmart.com	None	Static	Large	Depends on Software Purchased	Nondedicated	Keyboard Text to Speech	Direct Selection	Yes	Limited	No
Dec-Aid Adaptivation, Inc. 800–723–2783 www.adaptivation.com	Digitized	Static	Limited	None	Dedicated	Flexible Symbol Set	Direct Selection with Adaptivation's Pal Pads	Yes	Limited	No
DigiCom 2000 The Great Talking Box 408–456–0133 www.greattalking-box.com	Digitized	Static	Large	Levels	Dedicated	Flexible Symbol Set	Multiple Access Method Auditory Scan	Yes	Varied	No

(continues)

245

Table 9.4

(continued)

AAC Device	Voice Output	Display	Vocabulary Size	Vocabulary Expansion	Type of System	Symbol Type	Access Method	Portable/ Light-weight	Symbol Grid	ECU
Dubby TASH 800–463–5685 www.tashinc.com	Synthesized	Static	Large	Word Prediction	Dedicated	Keyboard with Text to Speech	Direct Selection	Yes	Limited	No
Dynamic Talk Back 27 Crestwood Communication Aids, Inc. 414–352–5678 www.communicationaids.com	Digitized	Static	Limited	Levels	Dedicated	Flexible Symbol Set	Direct Selection	Yes	Limited	No
Dynamo DynaVox, A Division of Sunrise Medical 888–697–7332 www.dynavoxsys.com	Digitized	Black-and-White Dynamic	Large	Page Linking	Dedicated	Flexible Symbol System	Multiple Access Methods Auditory Prompts	Yes	Varied	Yes
DynaMyte 3100 DynaVox, A Division of Sunrise Medical 888–697–7332 www.dynavoxsys.com	Synthesized Limited Digitized	Color Dynamic	Large	Abbreviated Expansion Word Prediction Page Linking	Dedicated	Flexible Symbol Set	Multiple Access Methods Auditory Prompts	Yes	Adjustable	Yes

Device	Speech	Display	Size	Rate Enhancement	Vocabulary	Symbol/Keyboard	Access		Adjustable	
DynaVox 3100 DynaVox, A Division of Sunrise Medical 888–697–7332 www.dynavoxsys.com	Synthesized Limited Digitized	Color Dynamic	Large	Abbreviated Expansion Word Prediction Page Linking	Dedicated	Flexible Symbol Set	Multiple Access Methods Auditory Prompts	No	Adjustable	Yes
DynaWrite DynaVox, A Division of Sunrise Medical 888–697–7332 www.dynavoxsys.com	Synthesized	Static	Large	Abbreviated Expansion Word Prediction	Dedicated	Keyboard with Text to Speech	Direct Selection	Yes	Limited	Yes
DynaWrite with Scanning Overlay DynaVox, A Division of Sunrise Medical 888–697–7332 www.dynavoxsys.com	Synthesized	Static	Large	Abbreviated Expansion Word Prediction	Dedicated	Keyboard with Text to Speech	Scan	Yes	Limited	Yes
Easy Talk, ACCI The Great Talking Box 408–456–0133 www.greattalking-box.com	Digitized	Static	Large	Levels	Dedicated	Flexible Symbol Set	Multiple Access Methods	Yes	Varied	No

(continues)

Table 9.4

(continued)

AAC Device	Voice Output	Display	Vocabulary Size	Vocabulary Expansion	Type of System	Symbol Type	Access Method	Portable/ Light-weight	Symbol Grid	ECU
E-Talk The Great Talking Box 408–456–0133 www.greattalking-box.com	Synthesized Digitized	Color Dynamic	Large	Page Linking Text to Speech	Dedicated	Flexible Symbol Set	Multiple Access Methods	Yes	Adjustable	No
Five Compartments Series: Switch Only Enabling Devices 800–832–8697 www.enablingdevices.com	None	Static	Limited	None	Dedicated	Flexible Symbol Set	Scan	Yes	Limited	No
Five Compartments Series: Lights and Sounds, Sounds Only, Lights Only Enabling Devices 800–832–8697 www.enablingdevices.com	Digitized	Static	Limited	None	Dedicated	Flexible Symbol Set	Direct Selection	Yes	Limited	No
Four Compartments, Speech and Lights Enabling Devices 800–832–8697 www.enablingdevices.com	Digitized	Static	Limited	None	Dedicated	Flexible Symbol Set	Direct Selection	Yes	Limited	No

Device	Speech	Display	Vocabulary	Rate Enhancement	Dedicated	Symbol Set	Access			
Four Frame Talker Attainment Company www.attainmentcompany.com 800-327-4269	Digitized	Static	Limited	None	Nondedicated	Flexible Symbol Set	Direct Selection	Yes	Limited	No
Freedom 2000, Freedom 2000 LITE P Series, Freedom 2000, Toughbook, Freedom 2000 Extreme Toughbook Words + 800-869-8521 www.words-plus.com	Synthesized	Color Dynamic	Large	Page Linking Word Prediction	Nondedicated	Flexible Symbol Set	Multiple Access Methods	Yes, except for Freedom 2000	Adjustable	Yes
Full Moon Talker ERI 516-501-0235 www.eridevices.com	Digitized	Static	Limited	None	Dedicated	Flexible Symbol Set	Direct Selection	Yes	Limited	No
Gemini[c] Assistive Technology 800-793-9227 www.assistivetech.com	Synthesized Limited Digitized	Color Dynamic	Large	Page Linking	Nondedicated	Flexible Symbol Set	Multiple Access Methods	No	Adjustable	Yes
Gemini SE Assistive Technology 800-793-9227 www.assistivetech.com	Synthsized Limited Digitized	Color Dynamic	Large	Page Linking	Dedicated	Flexible Symbol Set	Multiple Access Methods	No	Adjustable	Yes

(continues)

Table 9.4

(*continued*)

AAC Device	Voice Output	Display	Vocabulary Size	Vocabulary Expansion	Type of System	Symbol Type	Access Method	Portable/ Light-weight	Symbol Grid	ECU
GO! Board Series: **Choo-Choo Train Go! Board, Passenger Car Pete, Go! Board, Caboose Go! Board, Teddy the Tug Go! Board, Schoolhouse Go! Board, Double Decker Go! Board, School Bus Go! Board, Skyscaper Go! Board** Enabling Devices 800–832–8697 www.enablingdevices.com	Digitized	Static	Limited	None	Dedicated	Flexible Symbol Set	Direct Selection	Yes	Limited	No
Go! Board with 4 Icon Holders, Go! Board with 6 Icon Holders, Go! Board with 8 Icon Holders Enabling Devices 800–832–8697 www.enablingdevices.com	Digitized	Static	Limited	None	Dedicated	Flexible Symbol Set	Direct Selection	Yes	Limited	No

Product	Output	Display	Size	Features	Type	Symbol	Access Method			
Go Talk Attainment Company 800-327-4269 www.attainmentcompany.com	Digitized	Static	Medium	Levels	Dedicated	Flexible Symbol Set	Direct Selection	Yes	Limited	No
Go Talk 4 Attainment Company 800-327-4269 www.attainmentcompany.com	Digitized	Static	Limited	Levels	Dedicated	Flexible Symbol Set	Direct Selection	Yes	Limited	No
Grooved Platform Communicator Enabling Devices 800-832-8697 www.enablingdevices.com	Digitized	Static	Limited	None	Dedicated	Flexible Symbol Set	Direct Selection	No	Limited	No
HandHeld, HandHeld EX (dedicated version) Enkidu Research, Inc. 716-352-0507 www.enkidu.net	Synthesized Digitized	Dynamic and Static	Large	Page Linking Word Prediction	Nondedicated	Flexible Symbol Set	Multiple Access Method	Yes	Varied	No
Hawk Adam Lab 734-334-1610 www.adamlab.com	Digitized	Static	Limited	None	Dedicated	Flexible Symbol Set	Direct Selection	Yes	Limited	No
Hawk II, Hawk III Adam Lab 734-334-1610 www.adamlab.com	Digitized	Static	Limited	Levels	Dedicated	Flexible Symbol Set	Direct Selection Jacks	Yes	Limited	No

(continues)

251

Table 9.4

(*continued*)

AAC Device	Voice Output	Display	Vocabulary Size	Vocabulary Expansion	Type of System	Symbol Type	Access Method	Portable/ Light-weight	Symbol Grid	ECU
Hip Talk Plus Enabling Devices 800–832–8697 www.enablingdevices.com	Digitized	Static	Limited	None	Dedicated	Flexible Symbol Set	Direct Selection	Yes	Limited	No
Hip Talk Series: One Message Hip Talk, Two Message Hip Talk, Four Message Hip Talk, Ten Message Hip Talk, Sixteen Message Hip Talk Enabling Devices 800–832–8697 www.enablingdevices.com	Digitized	Static	Limited	None	Dedicated	Flexible Symbol Set	Direct Selection	Yes	Limited	No
Hip-Step Talker Enabling Devices 800–832–8697 www.enablingdevices.com	Digitized	Static	Limited	None	Dedicated	Flexible Symbol Set	Direct Selection	Yes	Limited	No
iTalk2 Communicator Ablenet 800–322–0956 www.ablenetinc.com	Digitized	Static	Limited	None	Dedicated	Flexible Symbol Set	Direct Selection	Yes	Limited	No

Device / Manufacturer	Synthesized/Digitized	Static	Memory	Features	Type	Output	Access Method			
Light Writer Series: SL35, SL5, SL20/21, SL35/Cherry, SL35/Big Keys, SL55, SL56 ZYGO Industries, Inc. 800-234-6006 www.zygo-usa.com	Synthesized	Static	Large	Word Prediction Abbreviation Expansion Memory Keys	Dedicated	Keyboard with Text to Speech		Yes	Limited	No
Lighthawk Adam Lab 734-334-1610 www.adamlab.com	Digitized	Static	Limited	Levels	Dedicated	Flexible Symbol Set	Scan Mode	Yes	Limited	No
Link Assistive Technology 800-793-9227 www.assistivetech.com	Synthesized	Static	Large	Abbreviated Expansion Word Prediction Memory Keys	Dedicated	Keyboard with Text to Speech	Direct Selection	Yes	Limited	No
MaCaw ZYGO Industries, Inc. 800-234-6006 www.zygo-usa.com	Digitized	Static	Large	Levels	Dedicated	Flexible Symbol Set	Multiple Access Methods	Yes	Variety	No
Maxx II Crestwood Company 414-352-5678 www.communicationaids.com	Synthesized	Static	Large	Memory Keys	Dedicated	Keyboard with Text to Speech	Direct Selection	Yes	Limited	No

(continues)

253

Table 9.4
(*continued*)

AAC Device	Voice Output	Display	Vocabulary Size	Vocabulary Expansion	Type of System	Symbol Type	Access Method	Portable/Lightweight	Symbol Grid	ECU
Mayer-Johnson Hand Held Voice (R) Ability Research, Inc. 952-939-0121 www.skypoint.com/~ability/hhv.html	Digitized	Monochrome Dynamic	Large	Page Linking	Dedicated	Mayer-Johnson Symbol Set Only	Direct Selection	Yes	Adjustable	No
Mercury PC[c] Assistive Technology 800-793-9227 www.assistivetech.com	Synthesized Limited Digitized	Color Dynamic	Large	Page Linking	Nondedicated	Flexible Symbol Set	Multiple Access Methods	No	Adjustable	Yes
Mercury SE Assistive Technology 800-793-9227 www.assistivetech.com	Synthesized Limited Digitized	Color Dynamic	Large	Page Linking	Dedicated	Flexible Symbol Set	Multiple Access Methods	No	Adjustable	Yes
Message Box Satillo Corp. 330-674-6722 www.saltillo.com	Synthesized Limited Digitized	Static	Limited	None	Dedicated	Flexible Symbol Set	Direct Selection	Yes	Limited	No
MessageMate 40, MessageMate 20 Words + 800-869-8521 www.words-plus.com	Digitized	Static	Medium	None	Dedicated	Flexible Symbol Set	Multiple Access Methods	Yes	Limited	No

(continues)

Device / Contact										
Millenium PC[c] Speak With Us 888–203–3646 www.speakwithus.com	Synthesized	Color Dynamic	Large	Page Linking	Nondedicated	Flexible Symbol Set	Multiple Access Methods	No	Adjustable	Yes
Mini Mate Words + 800–869–8521 www.words-plus.com	Digitized	Static	Limited	None	Dedicated	Flexible Symbol Set	Multiple Access Methods	Yes	Varied	No
Mini MessageMate Words + 800–869–8521 www.words-plus.com	Digitized	Static	Limited	None	Dedicated	Flexible Symbol Set	Direct Selection	Yes	Limited	No
Mini-Com Enabling Devices 800–832–8697 www.enablingdevices.com	Digitized	Static	Limited	None	Dedicated	Flexible Symbol Set	Direct Selection	Yes	Limited	No
Motion Talker Enabling Devices 800–832–8697 www.enablingdevices.com	Digitized	Static	Limited	None	Dedicated	Flexible Symbol Set	Direct Selection	Yes	Limited	No
Multi-Level MessageMate 40 Words + 800–869–8521 www.words-plus.com	Digitized	Static	Large	Levels	Dedicated	Flexible Symbol Set	Multiple Access Methods	Yes	Limited	No
One by Four Talker Attainment Company 800–327–4269 www.attainmentcompany.com	Digitized	Static	Limited	None	Dedicated	Flexible Symbol Set	Direct Selection	Yes	Limited	No

Table 9.4

(continued)

AAC Device	Voice Output	Display	Vocabulary Size	Vocabulary Expansion	Type of System	Symbol Type	Access Method	Portable/ Light-weight	Symbol Grid	ECU
One-Step Communicator Ablenet 800-327-4269 www.attainmentcompany.com	Digitized	Static	Limited	None	Dedicated	Flexible Symbol Set	Direct Selection Switch Access	Yes	Limited	No
One Talker Attainment Company 800-322-0956 www.ablenetinc.com	Digitized	No Display	Limited	None	Dedicated	None	Direct Selection	Yes	Limited	No
Optimist ZYGO Industries, Inc. 800-234-6006 www.zygo-usa.com	Synthesized	Color Dynamic	Large	Page Linking	Nondedicated	Flexible Symbol Set	Direct Selection	Yes	Adjustable	No
Palm Top, Palm Top EX (dedicated version) Enkidu Research, Inc. 716-352-0507 www.enkidu.net	Digitized	Color Dynamic	Large	Page Linking	Nondedicated	Flexible Symbol Set	Direct Selection	Yes	Varied	No

Device	Speech	Display	Vocabulary	Features	Dedicated/Nondedicated	Symbol Set	Access			
Partner/One, Partner One/Stepper, Partner/Two, Partner/Four ERI 516–501–0235 www.eridevices.com	Digitized	Static	Limited	None	Dedicated	Flexible Symbol Set	Direct Selection	Yes	Limited	No
Pathfinder Prentke Romich Co. 800–262–1933 www.prentrom.com	Synthesized Limited Digitized	Color Dynamic and static	Large	Word Prediction Predictive Selection Scanning Icon Prediction Semantic Compaction	Dedicated	Unity	Multiple Access Methods	Yes	Limited	No
Personal Talker Innocomp 800–382–8622 www.sayitall.com	Digitized	Static	Limited	None	Dedicated	Flexible Symbol Set	Direct Selection	Yes	Limited	No
Personal Talker Attainment Company 800–327–4269 www.attainmentcompany.com	Digitized	Static	Limited	None	Nondedicated	Flexible Symbol Set	Direct Selection	Yes	Limited	No

(continues)

257

Table 9.4

(continued)

AAC Device	Voice Output	Display	Vocabulary Size	Vocabulary Expansion	Type of System	Symbol Type	Access Method	Portable/ Light-weight	Symbol Grid	ECU
Pocket Communicator Gus Communications, Inc. 866-487-1006 www.gusinc.com	Synthesized Digitized	Color Dynamic	Large	Page Linking	Dedicated, Nondedicated (versions)	Flexible Symbol Set	Direct Selection	Yes	Adjustable	No
Pocket Go Talk Attainment Company 800-327-4269 www.attainmentcompany. com	Digitized	Static	Limited	Levels	Dedicated	Flexible Symbol Set	Multiple Access Methods	Yes	Limited	No
Quad Talk Crestwood Company 414-352-5678 www.communicationaids. com	None	Static	Limited	None	Dedicated	Flexible Symbol Set	Scan	No	Limited	No
Rocking Plate Talker, Twin Talker Enabling Devices 800-832-8697 www.enablingdevices.com	Digitized	Static	Limited	None	Dedicated	Flexible Symbol Set	Direct Selection	Yes	Limited	No

Product / Contact	Speech	Display	Vocabulary Size	Rate Enhancement	Type	Symbol/Output	Access Method			
Rocking Say It Play It Enabling Devices 800-832-8697 www.enablingdevices.com	Digitized	Static	Limited	None	Dedicated	Flexible Symbol Set	Direct Selection	Yes	Limited	No
Say It Simply Plus Innocomp 800-382-8622 www.sayitall.com	Synthesized	Static	Large	Levels	Dedicated	Flexible Symbol Set	Direct Selection	Yes	Varied	No
Scan-It-All Innocomp 800-382-8622 www.sayitall.com	Synthesized	Static	Large	Levels	Dedicated	Flexible Symbol Set	Multiple Access Methods	Yes	Varied	No
Scanning LightWriter Series: SL-86, SL-85, SL-35 ZYGO Industries, Inc. 800-234-6006 www.zygo-usa.com	Synthesized	Static	Large	Word Prediction Memory Keys Abbreviation Expansion	Dedicated	Keyboard Text to Speech	Scan	Yes	Limited	No
Sequencer Adaptivation, Inc. 605-335-4445 www.adaptivation.com	Digitized	Static	Limited	None	Dedicated	Flexible Symbol Set	Direct Selection Switch Access	Yes	Limited	No
Shadow Talker Enabling Devices 800-832-8697 www.enablingdevices.com	Digitized	Static	Limited	None	Dedicated	Flexible Symbol Set	Direct Selection	Yes	Limited	No

(continues)

Table 9.4

(*continued*)

AAC Device	Voice Output	Display	Vocabulary Size	Vocabulary Expansion	Type of System	Symbol Type	Access Method	Portable/ Light- weight	Symbol Grid	ECU
Side Kick Satillo Corp. 330-674-6722 www.saltillo.com	Digitized	Static	Large	Semantic Compac- tion	Dedicated	Flexible Symbol Set	Multiple Access Methods Auditory Scan	Yes	Limited	No
Side Swiping Communicator Enabling Devices 800-832-8697 www.enablingdevices.com	Digitized	Static	Limited	None	Dedicated	Flexible Symbol Set	Direct Selection	Yes	Limited	No
Single-Message Chatter Switch, Partner Two ERI 516-501-0235 www.eridevices.com	Digitized	Static	Limited	None	Dedicated	Flexible Symbol Set	Direct Selection Jacks	Yes	Limited	No
Speak Easy Ablenet 800-322-0956 www.ablenetinc.com	Digitized	Static	Limited	None	Dedicated	Flexible Symbol Set	Multiple Access Methods	Yes	Limited	No

Product									
Speaking Homework Wiz, Speaking Merriam-Webster Dictionary & Thesaurus, Speaking Merriam-Webster Collegiate Dictionary, Speaking Language Master, Speaking Language Master Special Edition, Speaking Spanish–English Dictionary Franklin Electronic Publishers 800-525-9673 www.franklin.com	Synthesized	Static	Large	None	Nondedicated	Keyboard with Text to Speech	Direct Selection	Yes	Limited	No
Speaking Speller Crestwood Communication Aids, Inc. 414-352-5678 www.communicationaids.com	Synthesized	Static	Large	None	Nondedicated	Keyboard with Text to Speech	Direct Selection	Yes	Limited	No
Speech Therapist with Mirror Enabling Devices 800-832-8697 www.enablingdevices.com	Digitized	Static	Limited	None	Dedicated	Flexible Symbol Set	Direct Selection	Yes	Limited	No

(continues)

Table 9.4

(*continued*)

AAC Device	Voice Output	Display	Vocabulary Size	Vocabulary Expansion	Type of System	Symbol Type	Access Method	Portable/ Light-weight	Symbol Grid	ECU
Spelling Ace with Thesaurus, Spelling Corrector Plus, Homework Wiz Plus, Spanish–English Dictionary Franklin Electronic Publishers 800-525-9673 www.franklin.com	None	Static	Large	None	Nondedicated	Keyboard	Direct Selection	Yes	Limited	No
Step by Step Communicator Ablenet 800-322-0956 www.ablenetinc.com	Digitized	Static	Limited	None	Dedicated	Flexible Symbol Set	Direct Selection Switch Access	Yes	Limited	No
Step by Step Communicator with Levels Ablenet 800-322-0956 www.ablenetinc.com	Digitized	Static	Limited	Levels	Dedicated	Flexible Symbol Set	Direct Selection Switch Access	Yes	Limited	No
Super Hawk 6/12 Adam Lab 734-334-1610 www.adamlab.com	Digitized	Static	Medium	Levels	Dedicated	Flexible Symbol Set	Multiple Access Methods	Yes	Varied	No

Device				Levels						
Super Hawk Plus Adam Lab 734-334-1610 www.adamlab.com	Digitized	Static	Medium		Dedicated	Flexible Symbol Set	Multiple Access Methods Auditory Scan	Yes	Varied	No
Synergy Mac[c] Speak With Us 888-203-3646 www.speakwithus.com	Synthesized	Color Dynamic	Large	Page Linking	Nondedicated	Flexible Symbol Set	Multiple Access Methods	Yes	Adjustable	Yes
Tablet, Tablet EX (dedicated version) Enkidu Research, Inc. 716-352-0507 www.enkidu.net	Synthesized	Dynamic	Large	Page Linking Word Prediction	Nondedicated	Flexible Symbol Set	Multiple Access Method	Yes	Varied	No
Take N'Talk Series: Take or Place N'Talk, Group Take N' Talk, Group Take or Place N' Talk, Classroom Take N'Talk, Classroom Take or Place N' Talk, Take N' Talk Go! Board, Take or Place N' Talk Go! Board, Lapboard Take N' Talk, Lapboard Take or Place N' Talk Enabling Devices 800-832-8697 www.enablingdevices.com	Digitized	Static	Limited	None	Dedicated	Flexible Symbol Set	Direct Selection	No	Limited	No

(continues)

263

Table 9.4

(continued)

AAC Device	Voice Output	Display	Vocabulary Size	Vocabulary Expansion	Type of System	Symbol Type	Access Method	Portable/ Light-weight	Symbol Grid	ECU
Talk Back 24 Crestwood Company 414–352–5678 www.communicationaids.com	Digitized	Static	Limited	None	Dedicated	Flexible Symbol Set	Direct Selection	Yes	Limited	No
Talk Back 36 Crestwood Company 414–352–5678 www.communicationaids.com	Digitized	Static	Medium	None	Dedicated	Flexible Symbol Set	Direct Selection	Yes	Limited	No
Talk Back III Crestwood Company 414–352–5678 www.communicationaids.com	Digitized	Static	Limited	None	Dedicated	Flexible Symbol Set	Direct Selection	Yes	Limited	No
Talk Trac Plus Ablenet 800–322–0956 www.ablenetinc.com	Digitized	Static	Limited	None	Dedicated	Flexible Symbol Set	Direct Selection	Yes	Limited	No

Product									
Talk Trac Plus with Levels Ablenet 800-322-0956 www.ablenetinc.com	Digitized	Static	Limited	Levels	Dedicated	Flexible Symbol Set	Direct Selection	Yes	Limited	No
Talking Box Voice In Box Enabling Devices 800-832-8697 www.enablingdevices.com	Digitized	Static	Limited	None	Dedicated	Flexible Symbol Set	Switch Access	Yes	Limited	No
Talking Buddy Innocomp 800-382-8622 www.sayitall.com	Digitized	Static	Limited	None	Dedicated	Flexible Symbol Set	Direct Selection	Yes	Limited	No
Talking Crestalk-ABC Crestwood Communication Aids, Inc. 414-352-5678 www.communicationaids.com	Synthesized	Static	Large	None	Dedicated	Letters Only: No Text to Speech	Direct Selection	Yes	Limited	No

(continues)

Table 9.4

(*continued*)

AAC Device	Voice Output	Display	Vocabulary Size	Vocabulary Expansion	Type of System	Symbol Type	Access Method	Portable/ Light-weight	Symbol Grid	ECU
Talking Picture Card Holder Enabling Devices 800-832-8697 www.enablingdevices.com	Digitized	Static	Limited	None	Dedicated	Flexible Symbol Set	Direct Selection	Yes	Limited	No
Talking Switch Plate Enabling Devices 800-832-8697 www.enablingdevices.com	Digitized	Static	Limited	None	Dedicated	Flexible Symbol Set	Direct Selection	Yes	Limited	No
Tech Scan Plus AMDI 516-466-2288 www.amdi.net	Digitized	Static	Medium	Levels	Dedicated	Flexible Symbol Set	Multiple Access Methods Auditory Scan	Yes	Limited	No
Tech Talk, Tech II 8 AMDI 516-466-2288 www.amdi.net	Digitized	Static	Medium	Levels	Dedicated	Flexible Symbol Set	Direct Selection	Yes	Limited	No
Tech/Four AMDI 516-466-2288 www.amdi.net	Digitized	Static	Limited	None	Dedicated	Flexible Symbol Set	Direct Selection	Yes	Limited	No

Product										
Tech/Scan AMDI 516-466-2288 www.amdi.net	Digitized	Static	Medium	Levels	Dedicated	Flexible Symbol Set	Multiple Access Methods	Yes	Limited	No
Tech/Speak Tech II 32 AMDI 516-466-2288 www.amdi.net	Digitized	Static	Medium	Levels	Dedicated	Flexible Symbol Set	Multiple Access Methods	Yes	Limited	No
The ComBoard TASH 800-463-5685 www.tashinc.com	None	Static	Limited	None	Dedicated	Flexible Symbol Set	Scan	Yes	Adjustable	No
The Communication Station Innocomp 800-382-8622 www.sayitall.com	Synthesized	Color Dynamic	Large	Page Linking	Nondedicated	Flexible Symbol Set	Multiple Access Methods	Yes	Adjustable	No
Three Compartments Series: **Lights and Sounds,** **Sounds Only** Enabling Devices 800-832-8697 www.enablingdevices.com	None	Static	Limited	None	Dedicated	Flexible Symbol Set	Direct Selection	Yes	Limited	No

(continues)

Table 9.4

(continued)

AAC Device	Voice Output	Display	Vocabulary Size	Vocabulary Expansion	Type of System	Symbol Type	Access Method	Portable/ Light-weight	Symbol Grid	ECU
Three Compartments Speech and Lights Enabling Devices 800–832–8697 www.enablingdevices.com	Digitized	Static	Limited	None	Dedicated	Flexible Symbol Set	Direct Selection	Yes	Limited	No
Three Compartments Switch Only Enabling Devices 800–832–8697 www.enablingdevices.com	None	Static	Limited	None	Dedicated	Flexible Symbol Set	Scan	Yes	Limited	No
Touch Corder Soft Touch Inc. 877–763–8868 www.funsoftware.com	Digitized	Static	Limited	None	Dedicated	Flexible Symbol Set	Direct Selection	Yes	Limited	No
TufTalker, TufTalker Plus, TufTalker Plus (without touch screen) Words + 800–869–8521 www.words–plus.com	Synthesized	Color Dynamic	Large	Page Linking Word Prediction	Nondedicated	Flexible	Multiple Access Method	Yes	Adjustable	Yes

Product									
Twin Talk Series Enabling Devices 800–832–8697 www.enablingdevices.com	Digitized	Static	Limited	None	Dedicated	Flexible Symbol Set	Direct Selection	Yes	Limited	No
Two Compartments Series: Lights and Sounds, Sounds Only Enabling Devices 800–832–8697 www.enablingdevices.com	None	Static	Limited	None	Dedicated	Flexible Symbol Set	Direct Selection	Yes	Limited	No
Two Compartments Speech and Lights Enabling Devices 800–832–8697 www.enablingdevices.com	Digitized	Static	Limited	None	Dedicated	Flexible Symbol Set	Direct Selection	Yes	Limited	No
Two Compartments Switch Only Enabling Devices 800–832–8697 www.enablingdevices.com	None	Static	Limited	None	Dedicated	Flexible Symbol Set	Scan	Yes	Limited	No
Ultimate TASH 800–463–5685 www.tashinc.com	Digitized	Static	Limited	None	Dedicated	Flexible Symbol Set	Direct Selection	Yes	Limited	No
Ultimate 8 TASH 800–463–5685 www.tashinc.com	Digitized	Static	Limited	None	Dedicated	Flexible Symbol Set	Direct Selection	Yes	Limited	No

(continues)

Table 9.4

(continued)

AAC Device	Voice Output	Display	Vocabulary Size	Vocabulary Expansion	Type of System	Symbol Type	Access Method	Portable/Light-weight	Symbol Grid	ECU
Vanguard Prentke Romich Co. 800-262-1933 www.prentrom.com	Synthesized Limited Digitized	Color Dynamic	Large	Word Prediction Predictive Selection Scanning Icon Prediction	Dedicated	Unity	Multiple Access Methods	No	Varied	No
VocaFlex Satillo Corp. 330-674-6722 www.saltillo.com	Digitized	Static	Large	Levels	Dedicated	Flexible Symbol Set	Direct Selection	Yes	Limited	No
Voice Mate TASH 800-463-5685 www.tashinc.com	Digitized	Static	Limited	None	Dedicated	Flexible Symbol Set	Direct Selection or Scan Model	Yes	Limited	No
VoicePal Max Adaptivation, Inc. 605-335-4445 www.adaptivation.com	Digitized	Static	Limited	None	Dedicated	Flexible Symbol Set	Multiple Access Methods	Yes	Varied	No

Device									
VoicePal 8 Adaptivation, Inc. 605–335–4445 www.adaptivation.com	Digitized	Static	Limited	None	Dedicated	Flexible Symbol Set	Direct Selection with Taction Pads	Yes	Limited	No
VoicePal 8K Adaptivation, Inc. 605–335–4445 www.adaptivation.com	Digitized	Static	Limited	None	Dedicated	Flexible Symbol Set	Direct Selection	Yes	Limited	No
VoicePal Pro Adaptivation, Inc. 605–335–4445 www.adaptivation.com	Digitized	Static	Limited	None	Dedicated	Flexible Symbol Set	Direct Selection	Yes	Varied	No
XyberKids Pack[c] Xybernaut Solutions, Inc. 888–992–3777 www.xybernaut.com	Synthesized	Color Dynamic	Large	Page Linking	Nondedicated	Flexible Symbol Set	Direct Selection	Yes	Adjustable	No
Yes–No Talker + Crestwood Communication Aids, Inc. 414–352–5678 www.communicationaids.com	Synthesized Limited Digitized	Static	Limited	None	Dedicated	Flexible Symbol Set	Direct Selection	Yes	Limited	No

Note: The electronic communication devices listed in this chart are currently available in the New York City area as of November, 2002. (Due to the large number of commercially available electronic AAC devices, this is not a comprehensive listing). Electronic communication devices may contain features that are not represented in this chart.

Display

Electronic communication devices typically have a visual display. These displays may be in black and white or in color and may be static or dynamic. A static display consists of a finite number of locations representing the symbol grid. For example, a keyboard has a static display of 26 letters, a space bar, the numbers 0 through 9, and function keys (e.g., backspace or delete word). Sometimes a static display is permanent; for example, the keyboard is the static display of a typewriter. Other times, a static display is set up so that different communication overlays (i.e., communication boards) can be placed on it to change the vocabulary items presented to the AAC user. A dynamic display looks like a computer screen. Computers allow the user to open different windows and get to new information within the parameters of the computer screen. Similarly, AAC devices with dynamic displays have a vocabulary expansion technique called page linking in which different communication pages open up when certain selections are made. Because communication overlays or boards are programmed into the device and change automatically, there is no need for paper overlays as with static displays. This allows increased vocabulary to be stored in these devices without the burden of carrying or changing communication overlays.

A few electronic devices have split screens, such that one portion is static and one portion is dynamic. Some electronic devices, whether they contain static or electronic displays, have various symbol grids. These grids can be interchanged on the device to change the number and size of the vocabulary items presented to the AAC user. The symbol grid on dynamic systems may be adjustable so that one can design a symbol grid configuration to accommodate the AAC user's needs and skills.

Output

All electronic communication devices have some sort of output, whether it is visual, print, audio, voice, or a combination of these. Visual output is usually presented in the form of a display with pictures or symbols, letters, words, phrases, or sentences that appear after and represent the selection. Sometimes visual cues are used to indicate that a selection has been made; these cues may simply be a light or arrow on the vocabulary item. Some devices have built-in printers or can be connected to a printer to produce written communication. Other electronic devices may have audio output (i.e., sounds such as a buzz, a beep, or a bell) to indicate that the AAC user has made a selection.

Speech output is a popular feature of electronic AAC systems. Voice output communication systems contain either synthesized or digitized speech that *speaks* the vocabulary item chosen. Synthesized speech refers to a computer-generated voice like the speech on your computer. Digitized speech is recorded speech similar to a tape recording: you just press a button to record your own voice into these devices. Different AAC systems will produce voice output at different times. Some give the user the ability to *speak* selection by selection (e.g., letter or picture symbols), others *speak* at the end of a word, some *speak* once punctuation has been added (the end of a sentence), and others give multiple options for when they will produce voice output. Many AAC systems give the user the opportunity to produce a message through the combination of multiple selections before the message is *spoken*. Once the formulation of the message (e.g., sentence) is finished, there are different ways for it to be spoken in its entirety. Some systems may have a "speak" button, whereas others produce voice output when the visual display (i.e., where the selected vocabulary items are displayed) is selected.

Some electronic devices contain keyboards. For some keyboards, when letters are selected to produce words, these words are *spoken* letter by letter. For example, the voice output of the written word "cat" would be pronounced "c" "a" "t." Most keyboards have a feature that is called *text to speech*. When written words are produced with this feature, the letters are translated into sounds, which are based on a specific language's grammatical rules, to produce words when spoken. For example, the voice output of the written word cat would be pronounced "cat."

Dedicated versus Nondedicated

Electronic communication devices are divided into two categories: dedicated and nondedicated devices. Dedicated devices are those electronic devices that were designed for the purpose of communication. Nondedicated devices are those that were not originally designed for communication purposes, such as a Spanish/English dictionary or a basic computer. These electronic devices are used for various purposes, only one of which is communication. A nondedicated, computer-based system allows the AAC user to have a full functioning computer and a complete communication system. When a computer-based system is used, separate communication software is sometimes required to enable the computer to be used as a communication system.

Many commercially available, ready-to-use application programs provide preprogrammed vocabulary pages to enhance language, increase conversational skills, and facilitate the construction of novel utterances in a quick and efficient manner. Some software programs may be available within dedicated devices (e.g., Unity is only available in Prentke Romich Company devices) (Badman et al., 1995). Other software programs may be used in a computer to enable it to function as a communication system. A variety of these application programs to match the AAC user's specific needs are commercially available. For example, some are picture symbol based, whereas others are word and letter based.

Environmental Control Units

Some electronic communication systems also have an environmental control unit (ECU) built in. The ECU enables the AAC user to control some electrical-based appliances in his or her environment (e.g., turn on lights or change channels on the television). ECUs can be infrared based or use a module that interrupts electricity flow.

Lightweight and Portable

Some electronic communication devices may be lightweight and portable to accommodate the needs of an ambulatory AAC user. Other communication devices may be big and heavy and are best suited for mounting on a wheelchair, walker, stroller, or table.

DETERMINING THE APPROPRIATENESS OF AN AUGMENTATIVE AND ALTERNATIVE COMMUNICATION SYSTEM

Because various AAC systems are available, a full comprehensive evaluation should be performed to determine the appropriateness of an AAC system for a specific individual and his or her communication needs and skills. A certified speech-language pathologist who specializes in augmentative and alternative communication (often called an *augmentative and alternative communication specialist*) should perform this evaluation. An AAC evaluation usually begins with obtaining background information on the individual before the actual evaluation. This background information may be provided through preassessment forms; an interview with a social worker, case manager, or client coordinator; reports from specialists in various disciplines (speech, occupational, and physical therapists; psychologists, psychiatrists, audiologists, vision specialists, medical personnel, and educational personnel); and information provided by family members and support staff (i.e., aides, residential staff, and nursing staff). Background information should include the diagnosis and its future impact upon the individual and his or her skills (i.e., progressive versus static disorder, temporary versus permanent disorder, sensory skills, physical status, and cognitive and language skills), communication needs, previous success and failure with AAC, methods of access that have been previously used or are presently being used, and educational or work-related status and goals. This information will enable the augmentative and alternative communication Specialist to be better prepared to determine which AAC system will best meet the needs and skills of the individual.

During the evaluation process, the augmentative and alternative communication specialist may ask for support from the following professionals to aid in the evaluation process: occupational therapist, physical therapist or seating specialist, rehabilitation engineer, vision specialist, psychologist, teacher, and job trainer. Various evaluative tasks should be performed to assess the individual's current language skills, cognitive skills, auditory skills, and vision and motor and positioning status as they pertain to the design and use of an AAC system. Tasks within the evaluation should also include trial use of different AAC systems.

It is important to look at the AAC user as a "whole" person with many different strengths and weaknesses, who communicates with various partners who also have different strengths and weaknesses, and who communicates in various environments that may or may not foster easy communication. Communication is performed within an environment and with at least one communication partner. Therefore information about the user's environment (i.e., with whom the individual will communicate, where will the individual communicate, and what will the individual need to communicate) needs to be compiled during the evaluation. The user's needs and the communication partner's needs and skills will determine the design of the AAC system. For example, if the listener does not read, then the AAC user will need either a voice output system or a system that contains a symbol set that the communication partner recognizes. If the communication partner speaks a different language than the AAC user, then the communication system needs to contain vocabulary in both languages so that both the user and listener will be able to communicate together. Specific details about the environments in which the communication interactions will take place need to be considered, because they have an impact on the design of the AAC system. For example, if the AAC user is going to communicate in an extremely noisy environment with partners in various positions within that environment, then the AAC system should include voice output with adjustable volume.

Once the individual's skills, status, and communication needs (i.e., user needs, partner needs, and environmental obstacles) are determined, they can now be matched to an AAC system. AAC systems should always be modified to the user's specific needs and skills. The user should not adapt to the AAC system. For example, if an individual is on an object level, the recommended AAC system should permit the use of objects as its symbol set, so it can be used when it is received. The system should not contain only picture symbols, which require the AAC user to further develop his or her cognitive skills before using the AAC system. During the evaluation it should be determined whether a manual or electronic system or both are needed. When an electronic communication system is recommended, the user's skills should be closely matched to the features provided by the electronic device to promote optimal communication. For example, if an individual has a progressive neurologic disorder, then the electronic device should include scanning options in addition to direct selection, because the user's physical status will deteriorate over time, which may result in direct selection no longer being a viable option.

Once a manual system or electronic device is chosen, then the augmentative and alternative communication specialist needs to determine whether any accessories will be needed to optimize the use of the AAC system. Accessories to facilitate functional use of the manual system or electronic device may include mounting systems, an access method (i.e., a switch), keyguards, a communication software program, speakers, and a carrying case. After choosing an AAC system, the augmentative and alternative communication specialist needs to decide whether the system should be rented or purchased. If the specialist decides that the AAC user needs a trial period to assess his or her functional use of the system or needs training to determine the appropriateness of the system (e.g., for further assessment of switch use related to accuracy and fatigue), then the AAC system should be rented for a period. If the augmentative and alternative communication specialist is confident that the AAC user demonstrates functional use of the recommended AAC system, then its purchase should be pursued through the individual's funding source. After the evaluation, a report that describes the evaluation and the recommended equipment should be written and submitted to the individual's funding source for rental or purchase of the AAC system.

When an AAC system is chosen, it is considered optimal for the individual's current status and the technology available at the time. It is important to realize that nothing in the AAC user's life or with technology remains stagnant. An individual's skills or communication needs may change over time. These changes may be attributed to diagnosis, improvement in skills due to training, aging or developmental issues, or acquisition of a job, to list just a few. As these changes occur it may be necessary to modify or completely change his or her AAC system. Advancements in available technologies are another reason that a user's AAC system may be altered. Therefore it is important that reassessments be done periodically to determine the continued appropriateness of an AAC system. They should be done as the user's skills or communication needs change and when new technologies that may improve the effectiveness of the AAC system become available.

FUNDING

There are many sources for the funding of AAC systems. Different states have different funding guidelines. Typically, AAC systems may be funded through educational, medical, vocational, and private sources. Educational funding sources may include early intervention programs and school district or board of education support to provide children younger than age 21 years with improved communication in the classroom. Medical sources may include Medicaid, Medicare, and general health insurance companies that provide AAC systems to individuals who require a better way to communicate their medical needs. Vocational funding sources in New York include Vocational Educational Services for Individuals with Disabilities (VESID), which provide AAC systems to those who require them to be able to gain employment. Private funding sources, such as religious organizations, group rallies, company donations, and private payers, may also provide assistance to gain AAC systems. All evaluations for AAC systems should reflect the particular goals of the specific funding source. For example, when funding through a medical insurance company is sought, the medical necessity for the AAC system must be demonstrated.

TRAINING

Once an AAC evaluation is completed, and it is determined that an AAC system is warranted, then training should begin. If the individual does not demonstrate the basic requirements for an AAC system, then the required prerequisites should be taught. Included are cognitive, receptive language, and access skills. Instruction may be needed for developing object permanence or moving the individual through the symbol set hierarchy from object to picture symbols within structured activities. Switch use may need to be practiced through the use of switch toys, computer software programs, or electronic communication devices. Communication intent may also need to be facilitated during various communicative environments through role-playing activities.

Once an AAC system is chosen, setup and training should begin. Setup includes vocabulary analysis, the design and production of a manual communication system, the organization and programming of vocabulary items into an electronic communication device, and the placement or mounting of the various components of the AAC system. To ensure its functional use the user's visual, auditory, and physical status must be taken into account. The arrangement of manual communication systems, electronic communication devices, switches, and other accessories should be done with great care and attention. Placement or mounting issues may include the need for the AAC system to be on an angle to facilitate ease of access or visual attending. If an individual is right-handed and cannot cross the midline, then the switch or communication system should be made accessible by placement to the right of the midline. If an individual is using auditory prompts and is hearing impaired, then the speaker must be placed next to the ear with the best residual hearing.

Once the AAC is set up, training is required to optimize efficient use of it across all environments. Teaching is needed for all AAC systems, regardless of the level of complexity of the system. Instruction may entail helping family members or support staff become comfortable with the daily setup and breakdown of the AAC system, learning basic maintenance of the manual communication system or electronic device, training on vocabulary retrieval, practicing of scanning skills, and facilitating functional use of the AAC system. Often, training is initially needed to reinforce the individual's use of his or her AAC system instead of previously used communication modes. The individual with a hearing impairment who signed in all environments may require prompts to communicate using his or her communication system with communication partners who do not understand sign language.

Within training techniques, there is a hierarchy of facilitative cues. They include imitation, models, prompts, and role-playing activities. Prompts that are used may be verbal, visual, or tactile. All cues are important in the successful acquisition of a skill. To facilitate the use of an AAC system, the communication interaction must be designed to allow for its use. For instance, to foster the use of various vocabulary items the communication partner should use open-ended phrases, sentences, or questions as opposed to excessive use of yes or no questions. The listener should provide pauses or ample time for the AAC user to access his or her communication system. Too often, the communication partner is used to playing 20 questions or anticipating the user's response and does not allow him or her to respond. As a communication partner, one should not be afraid of silence. Often, the AAC user needs this time to make a vocabulary selection on his or her communication system. Another technique commonly used by a communication partner is doing something wrong in a particular situation (e.g., putting a shelled egg into the batter when baking) or doing something out of sequence (e.g., squeezing the tube of toothpaste before taking the cap off). Thus the AAC user has an opportunity to spontaneously use his or her communication system to correct the communication partner's action. This facilitates initiation of communication as well as commenting on and directing others, to name just a few pragmatic functions fostered by this technique.

The level of involvement of support from staff and family members will determine the success of the AAC user in use of his or her system across all environments. To encourage functional use of an AAC system, all communication partners must support its use in all environments. Therefore facilitative techniques from therapy sessions must be carried on by family members, support staff, and all other communication partners in all settings. Functional use requires that skills be learned in a lifelike, communicative-interaction atmosphere as opposed to a stale, instructional, teacher and student learning environment. For example, reviewing food vocabulary items and having the individual simply identify them does not mean that he or she will use them when at a restaurant. These vocabulary items will best be learned when the individual role-plays a restaurant activity. Therefore to encourage spontaneous use of an individual's AAC system, practice must occur within functional situations.

There are various commercially available training techniques that use different strategies to facilitate the use of AAC. These techniques may be designed for a specific group of individuals to foster skill development in different environments or for general training techniques to foster improved communication. For example, The Picture Exchange Communication System (PECS) (Frost & Bondy, 1994) was developed to train AAC to individuals with autism and others with socially inappropriate behaviors.

Various materials to facilitate AAC in different settings are available (Elder & Goosens, 1996; Goosens, Crain, & Elder, 1995). The individual's communication symbols should be readily available throughout his or her day in all environments. Communication displays or symbols should be seen and be easily accessible by the user for communication purposes. Communication partners should also have access to these displays or symbols for modeling and training purposes. During training stages, communication partners should use symbols when they speak to the user to stimulate and help facilitate the AAC user's knowledge of symbols.

SUMMARY

As discussed in this chapter, the goal of augmentative and alternative communication is to enable effective, quick, and accurate communication. Individuals with various disabilities can be assisted by the use of AAC techniques. Over the years, many changes have been seen in the field of AAC and many developments are yet to come. Language and cognitive skills and visual, auditory, and motor or positioning status play an important role in the design and use of AAC systems. The individual AAC user, support staff, and environments in which the AAC user will communicate further determine the most appropriate AAC system. An AAC system consists of a manual or electronic communication device and all of its accessories. Because various AAC systems are available, it is important that a comprehensive evaluation be performed to determine the optimal AAC system for an individual given his or her communication needs, skills, and communicative environments. This evaluation should be conducted by a speech-language pathologist who specializes in AAC, along with input from other professionals. There are different sources for the funding of AAC systems that vary from state to state.

Training should be provided before, during, and after the acquisition of the AAC system to ensure its functional use. There are various training techniques and commercially available instructional materials that use different strategies to facilitate the use of AAC systems. The level of involvement of support staff and family members determines the success of use of an AAC system across all environments. To encourage functional use of an AAC system, it is critical that it is used in all environments and supported by all communication partners. It is important to remember that as an individual's communicative needs or skills change over time, so should his or her AAC system.

REFERENCES

American Speech-Language-Hearing Association. (1989). Competencies for speech-language pathologists providing services in augmentative communication. *ASHA, 31*, 107–110.

American Speech-Language-Hearing Association. (1991). Report: Augmentative and alternative communication. *ASHA, 33*(Suppl. 5), 10.

Badman, A. L., Baker, B. R., Banajee, M., Cross, R. T., Lehr, J. S., Maro, J., et al. (1995). *Unity: A Minspeak application program.* Wooster, OH: Prentke Romich.

Baker, B. (1982). Minspeak. *Byte, 9,* 186–202.

Beukelman, D., Yorkston, K., & Dowden, P. (1985). *Communication augmentation: A casebook of clinical management* (p. 3). San Diego: College Hill Press.

Beukelman, D., & Mirenda, P. (1992). *Augmentative and alternative communication management of severe communication disorder in children and adults* (p. 59). Paul H. Brookes.

Cook, A., & Hussey, S. (1995). *Assistive technologies: Principles and practice* (pp. 14–19). St. Louis: Mosby-Yearbook.

Drinker, P. A., & Krupoff, S. (1981). Eye-link for non-vocal communication: Direct selection by eye contact. Paper presented at the Fourth Annual Conference on Rehabilitation Engineering, Washington, DC.

Elder, P., & Goosens, C. (1996). *Engineering training environments for interactive augmentative communication strategies for adolescents and adults who are moderately/severely developmentally delayed* (2nd rev. ed.). Birmingham: Southeast Augmentative Communication Conference Publications.

Frost, L., & Bondy, A. (1994). *PECS: The Picture Exchange Communication System training manual.* Cherry Hill, NJ: Pyramid Educational Consultants.

Goosens', C., Crain, S., & Elder, P. (1995). *Engineering the preschool environment for interactive symbolic communication 18 months to 5 years developmentally* (3rd ed.). Birmingham, AL: Southeast Augmentative Communication Conference.

Scholl, G. (1986). Visual impairment and other exceptionalities. In G. Scholl (Ed.), Foundations of education for blind and visually handicapped children and youth: Theory and practice (pp. 137–144). New York: American Foundation for the Blind.

Vanderheiden, G. C., & Lloyd, L. L. (1986). Communication systems and their components. In S. Blackstone, & D. Bruskin (Ed.), *Augmentative communication: An introduction.* Rockville, MD: American Speech-Language and Hearing Association.

SELECTED READINGS

Bain, B. K., & Leger, D. (Eds.). (1997). *Assistive technology: An interdisciplinary approach.* New York: Churchill Livingston.

Case-Smith, J. (2001). *Occupational therapy for children* (4th ed.). St. Louis: Mosby.

Connor, F., Williamson, G., & Siepp, J (Eds.). (1978). *Program guide for infants and toddlers with neuromuscular and other developmental disorders.* New York: Teacher College Press.

Domjan, M. & Burkhard, B. (1986). *The principles of learning & behavior* (2nd ed.). Pacific Grove, CA: Brooks/Cole.

Enders, A., & Hall, M. (Eds.). (1990). *Assistive technology sourcebook.* Washington, DC: RESNA.

Fishman, I. (1987). *Electronic communication aids selection and use.* Boston, MA: College-Hill.

Lahey, M. (1988). *Language disorders and language development* (rev. ed.). New York: Macmillan.

Mann, W., & Lane, J. (Eds.) (1993). The human face of AAC technology. In D. J. Higginbotham (Issue Ed.), *Technology and Disability, 2*(3).

Morris, D. (1993). *Dictionary of communication disorders* (2nd ed.). London: Whurr.

Trombly, C. A. (Ed.). (1989). *Occupational therapy for physical dysfunction* (3rd ed.). Baltimore: Williams & Wilkins.

CHAPTER 10

RESPECTFUL Counseling:
A Blueprint for Practice

Brenda Y. Cartwright, Ed.D., CRC, LPC
Department of Counselor Education
University of Hawaii at Manoa
Honolulu, HA

Individuals with Hearing Impairments
Facilitating Communication
RESPECTFUL Counseling Framework
    Religious/Spiritual Identity
    Economic Class Standing
    Sexual Identity
    Psychologic Maturity
    Ethnic/Racial Identity
    Chronologic/Developmental Challenges
    Trauma and Other Threats to One's Well-Being
    Family History and Influence
    Unique Physical Characteristics
    Location of Residence and Language Differences
Conclusion
References

Although counselors are committed to improving the quality of people's lives, an abundance of empirical research suggests ongoing disparities with the efficacy of treatment among individuals from diverse groups and backgrounds. The U.S. Surgeon General's Report (2001) clearly demonstrated that more persons of color (i.e., Native Americans,

African Americans, Latinos, and Asian/Pacific Islanders) than all other Americans are both underserved and ineffectively served by counselors and other mental health professionals.

The U.S. Surgeon General's Report (SGR) is particularly important for several reasons. First, it was published at a time in which the demography of the United States was undergoing unprecedented changes and people of color accounted for an increasing proportion of the nation's population. The changing complexion and diversification of our nation challenge many fundamental precepts from which counselors and other mental health professionals operate, typically from an ethnocentric monocultural perspective (Sue & Sue, 2003). This perspective is characterized by western European culture and class-based values with an emphasis on verbal communications and use of standard English. Yet researchers, educators, practitioners, and other counseling professionals are perplexed about the underutilization and premature termination of service in mental health agencies by people of color.

Second, the SGR challenges us to consider both our legal and ethical responsibilities when working with persons from diverse cultures and backgrounds. Legally, practitioners must adhere to applicable state laws and federal regulations. The codes of ethics of the American Counseling Association (1996), the American Psychological Association (2002), and the Commission on Rehabilitation Counselor Certification (2002) outlined practitioners' ethical responsibilities of (1) respect for all people, regardless of age, color, culture, disability, ethnic group, gender, religion, sexual orientation, marital status, or socioeconomic status and (2) obtaining competency in serving diverse groups of people. However, we must recognize that knowledge of the principles and guidelines promulgated by these codes does not automatically improve practitioners' sensitivity and effectiveness in working with persons from diverse groups and backgrounds. Research and clinical practice continue to propel practitioners to incorporate multicultural counseling competence in service provision to improve utilization and improve efficiency of treatment for individuals from diverse groups and backgrounds.

In addition, a review of the rehabilitation literature (Atkins & Wright, 1980; Bowe, 1984; Moore, 2001; Moore & Schroedel, 2001; Patterson, Allen, Parnell, Crawford, & Beardall, 2000; Wilson, 2002) underscores the SGR findings, which showed that counselors have not provided equitable services to clients from traditionally underrepresented groups from nonwhite populations and to persons from specific disability groups (e.g., individuals with hearing losses). Overall, these clients had less access to rehabilitation services and were less likely to receive needed care. When they received care, it was more likely to be poor in quality.

INDIVIDUALS WITH HEARING IMPAIRMENTS

With the aging process and increased exposure to noise, it is estimated that about 1 of 10 Americans is hearing impaired (U.S. Bureau of the Census, 2001). According to the National Institute on Deafness and Other Communication Disorders (NIDCD), more than 28 million persons in the U.S. population are deaf or hard of hearing, with the largest group (40%) including those who are elderly. Counselors will inevitably encounter individuals with hearing losses in general practice, particularly because having a hearing loss does not make them immune to other issues, not necessarily related to the hearing loss, that bring people to counseling. However, despite the growing incidence of Americans with hearing losses, most counseling practitioners are ill-prepared to assist these clients to improve the quality of their overall lifestyle for effective functioning in the workplace and in social and family contexts.

FACILITATING COMMUNICATION

Because each individual with a hearing loss is unique, having different experiences and communication needs, counselors are urged to make an initial assessment of the factors that contributed to its onset and the degree to which it impairs the client. During this assessment, attention should be focused on evaluating whether the hearing loss developed before language acquisition or later in adulthood. Those individuals with congenital or prelingual hearing losses, as a group, increasingly choose to eschew a disability identity and view themselves as a minority linguistic community, whereas those who acquired their loss adventitiously maintain their lives in the hearing community, relying on residual hearing and visual cues for communication (Robertson, 1999). The second and perhaps most important step in the counseling process with these clients is to determine how the individual prefers to communicate. Such preferences may include speech reading (formerly known as lip reading), sign language, writing, or any combination of these.

If the client can and prefers to speech read, face her or him directly when speaking. Use a natural tone and rhythm when speaking to the client; exaggerated pronunciation makes speech reading more difficult. Eating; chewing gum; placing one's hands over the mouth; having long hair, moustaches, or beards; looking down at notes or forms; or holding paper in front of the face when reading from them undermines counselors' ability to communicate effectively with these clients. It is helpful to remember that 40–60% of the English sounds appear the same on the lips. In fact, even the best speech readers in a one-to-one situation were found to understand only 26% of what was said to them (Mindel & Vernon, 1971, p. 96).

If the client uses American Sign Language, it is preferred that the counselor signs for herself or himself, but if this is not feasible, then a certified interpreter is the best communication facilitator. Counselors should not use family members or friends to help facilitate communication in counseling situations with these clients, because their emotional attachment to the client may influence *how* and *what* is conveyed. Interpreters are bound by a code of ethics to maintain confidentiality and to transmit accurate messages, without editing or adding their own opinions. In addition, counselors should not assume that because hearing co-workers know how to sign this is synonymous with knowing how to interpret. When using an interpreter, the counselor should address the client directly, "How are you?" not "How is he?" Regardless of whether the counselor is using speech only, signing for himself or herself, or using an interpreter, it is critical that the lips and facial expressions can be seen clearly by the hearing-impaired client.

If the client prefers writing, counselors should be sure to carefully evaluate the client's response to what he or she writes before continuing in the counseling session and gear all written materials to the client's level of understanding. Counselors are reminded that English is essentially a second language for many deaf clients; therefore words may be written in a different order or in what may be considered as incomplete sentences.

Practitioners in the fields of special education and rehabilitation suggest that because individuals with hearing losses rely on sight to obtain information, lighting and positioning must be considered to provide the best possible view of the speaker's face (Kampfe, 1990; Kampfe & Smith, 1999). The room should be well lit, with light on the face of the counselor. Care should be taken to ensure that counselors are not seated with their backs to the window, resulting in their faces being in a shadow. The close distance between the counselor and client may be a critical factor for the client to hear what is said.

In addition, extraneous sounds and room noises should be minimized. Background music designed for relaxation will possibly have the opposite effect on clients with hearing losses. The humming noises of fans, heaters, and air conditioners can interfere with communication, particularly if the client is using hearing aids that amplify the distracting noises.

The purpose of this chapter, therefore, is to increase counselors' awareness and knowledge for promotion of successful experiences with clients who have varying degrees and types of hearing losses and who simultaneously may come from culturally diverse groups and backgrounds. Particular attention will be directed to (1) the multidimensionality of clients' development and (2) the need for counselors to conduct a self-assessment about how varied historical-cultural-contextual factors have affected their own development. The counseling model that is presented in this chapter specifically focuses on a host of diversity and contextual issues that counselors are encouraged to consider as they strive to work more effectively, ethically, and respectfully with persons from diverse client populations, including those with hearing losses. Definitions of key terms and concepts included in this new counseling model are presented. A number of case scenarios demonstrate the practical utility of using this counseling framework to assess the client's and the counselor's multidimensionality. These scenarios (1) help the reader to better understand how the interaction of multiple factors in the RESPECTFUL counseling model might be manifested among clients with whom they work and (2) emphasize the need for counselors to continually assess the ways in which these multiple factors may have an impact on their own development and ways of approaching clients from diverse groups and backgrounds.

RESPECTFUL COUNSELING FRAMEWORK

The RESPECTFUL counseling model represents a new, comprehensive, and holistic approach to understanding how the client's and the counselor's multidimensionality affects the process and outcome of counseling. This includes (1) clients who seek professional assistance with various problems and challenges they are encountering in their lives and (2) mental health professionals (e.g., counselors, social workers, and psychologists) who are trained to assist clients to acquire the knowledge and skills that will enable them to lead more effective and satisfying lives.

Two theoretical assumptions underlie the foundation on which the RESPECTFUL counseling framework is based. The first assumption is based on the belief that the ultimate goal of all counseling is to promote clients' psychologic and personal development. Counselors routinely use their knowledge and skills to achieve this broad goal by

1. fostering the development of more effective decision-making and problem-solving competencies that can be used by clients who are not necessarily in crisis but are in need of acquiring more effective life skills,
2. providing crisis counseling services that are designed to help clients develop more effective coping strategies during times of heightened stress, and
3. using more intensive, long-term psychotherapeutic interventions that are aimed at stimulating qualitative changes in clients' personality development.

The second assumption that underlies the RESPECTFUL counseling model involves the importance of understanding the unique and complex multidimensionality of human development and the need to intentionally address the multiple factors that have an impact on clients' development in counseling practice. The counseling profession in general is beginning to demonstrate a greater awareness of the ways in which various cultural-contextual dimensions of a person's life affect his or her sense of psychologic well-being. The development of new theoretical insights and an abundance of research findings have helped mental health professionals reconstruct and expand their thinking about human development.

The RESPECTFUL counseling model addresses the multidimensionality of human development by directing attention to 10 factors that are known to have a significant impact on the psychologic development of both counselors and their clients. As will be discussed later in this chapter, this theoretical framework is useful to help counselors to (1) assess their own development, (2) identify their own cultural-contextual biases, (3) assess some of the factors that have an impact on their clients' development, and (4) understand how to more effectively and ethically address the interface of multiple cultural-contextual factors in counseling practice. The 10 factors that compose the RESPECTFUL counseling model include: *r*eligious/spiritual identity, *e*conomic class standing, *s*exual identity, *p*sychologic maturity, *e*thnic/racial identity, *c*hronologic/developmental challenges, *t*rauma and other threats to one's well-being, *f*amily history and influence, *u*nique physical characteristics, and *l*ocation of residence and language differences.

RELIGIOUS/SPIRITUAL IDENTITY

The first factor in the RESPECTFUL model focuses on the way in which individuals personally identify with established religions or hold beliefs about extraordinary experiences that go beyond the boundaries of the strictly objective, empirically perceived world that characterizes modern western psychologic thought (D'Andrea & Daniels, 2001). Kelly (1995) points out that the terms *religion* and *spirituality* are both grounded in an affirmation of transcendence or "otherness" that is typically manifested in religious forms that extend beyond the boundaries of the ordinary and tangible. As used in the RESPECTFUL counseling framework, religion and spirituality refer to a person's belief in a reality that transcends physical nature and provides individuals with an extraordinary meaning of life and human existence.

Although the terms *religion* and *spirituality* include the affirmation of a transcendental dimension of reality, they also have different meanings. As D'Andrea and Daniels (1997) explain:

> While the term spirituality is often used to refer to a person's belief and affirmation of a transcendental connectedness with the universe, religion is typically used to denote the specific ways in which the belief is manifested institutionally within the creeds and dogmas of different religious groups and denominations. As used in the RESPECTFUL counseling model, the term religious/spiritual identity refers to a person's beliefs about the afterlife and the interconnectedness of all things in the universe as well as one's views about the meaning of such concepts as "God," "enlightenment," and "grace" to name a few. (p. 30)

Because a client's religious/spiritual identity may play an important role in the way he or she constructs meaning of his or her life's experiences, it is important that early in the helping process counselors assess the degree to which this factor affects their client's psychologic development. It is equally important that counseling practitioners consider how their own religious/spiritual identity and beliefs may have a positive or negative impact on the work they do with clients who embrace different perspectives than their own. This is critical, because, when left unexamined, counselors' own religious/ spiritual identity and beliefs or lack thereof may result in inaccurate interpretations and misunderstandings of clients' development and their views about mental health and personal well-being (D'Andrea & Daniels, 1997).

ECONOMIC CLASS STANDING

Despite the tremendous impact that an individual's socioeconomic class standing has on his or her personal, psychologic, and career development, it is distressing to note how often counselors fail to consider this factor adequately when working with persons from diverse economic backgrounds. One of the reasons that many contemporary counseling practitioners fail to direct more attention to socioeconomic factors and their impact on human development lies in the overuse of terms that have little relevance in accurately describing many clients' economic group identities. The over-reliance on general categories, such as low, middle, and upper class backgrounds, represents an inadequate and, in many instances, an irrelevant way to describe this dimension of our clients' lives. To help counselors gain a greater understanding of the different economic classes or groups of which many clients are a part, D'Andrea and Daniels (2001) have extended the three general classes that social scientists traditionally have used to describe this variable by describing six socioeconomic classes or categories in which most persons in the United States can be classified. These researchers believe that this new classification system more accurately describes the different socioeconomic group identities that develop during the course of their lives.

This classification system includes (1) *poor persons*, unemployed individuals with less than a high school degree who are in need of economic assistance to meet their basic living needs; (2) *working poor persons*, individuals who have a high school or equivalency degree or some college experience, who are employed as unskilled workers, and whose annual incomes fall below the federal poverty guidelines; (3) *working class persons*, individuals who have a high school degree, have some college experience, or have received a certificate or license in a particular trade, whose annual incomes fall above the federal poverty guidelines; (4) *middle class nonprofessionals*, persons with at least a high school degree, but more likely with an advanced degree or specialized training in a given vocational career, whose annual incomes are above the national average; (5) *middle class professionals*, persons with at least a college degree, but more likely with an advanced degree in some professional field such as education, law, or medicine, whose annual incomes are above the national average; and (6) *persons in the upper class*, the smallest segment of persons whose annual incomes fall within the upper 10% of the national average.

A plethora of socioscientific research has focused on the ways in which people's economic class standing and background affect quality of life. To a large extent, this determines how long people live, whether they will have a healthy life, what the probability is that they will fail in school, and what types of employment outcomes they will experience in adulthood. Recognizing the influence that this aspect of clients' multidimensionality has on their development, practitioners must be attentive to the ways in which this factor contributes to an individual's identified strengths and expressed problems during counseling. Because counselors can easily develop inaccurate and negative views and prejudices about persons who come from economic backgrounds that are different from their own, it is important that these professionals evaluate their own class-based assumptions, biases, and stereotypes when working with individuals who come from diverse economic class groups.

SEXUAL IDENTITY

One of the most complex although often understudied aspects of an individual's psychologic development involves the sexual identity development of persons who come from diverse groups and backgrounds in our society. As used in the RESPECTFUL counseling model, the term *sexual identity* relates to a person's gender identity, gender roles, and sexual orientation. A brief discussion of these three components of people's sexual identity follows.

Gender identity refers to an individual's subjective sense of what it means to be either male or female. A person's gender identity is clearly affected by the different roles men and women are expected to play within a given cultural-ethnic context. Bailey (1996) notes that the type of gender identity that one develops is markedly influenced by "those behaviors, attitudes, and personality traits that a society designates as masculine or feminine, that is, more 'appropriate' for or typical of the male or female role" (p. 72).

A person's sexual identity can be manifested in ways that extend beyond the narrow notion of masculinity and femininity. For example, *transsexualism* refers to those persons who experience discordance between their gender identity and their anatomical sex, whereas *androgyny* refers to those individuals who manifest a combination of masculine and feminine traits and behaviors (Bailey, 1996).

A person's sexual identity is also influenced by his or her *sexual orientation.* There are a number of ways to conceptualize this dimension of a person's sexual identity. In general, this includes bisexuality, heterosexuality, and homosexuality. *Bisexuality* refers to individuals who demonstrate a sexual interest in both males and females. *Heterosexuality,* in contrast, refers to individuals whose sexual interest is directed toward persons of the opposite sex, and *homosexuality* refers to individuals whose sexual preference involves persons of the same sex.

In light of the negative stereotypes that have historically been associated with the term *homosexuality*, words such as gay males, gays, and lesbians are considered more acceptable and respectful terms to use to describe this dimension of a person's sexual identity (D'Andrea & Daniels, 2001). Counselors must recognize the important impact that clients' and practitioners' sexual identity has in counseling and psychotherapeutic settings and the tremendous impact that sexual identity issues may have on a person's psychologic development and sense of personal well-being.

Thus from the perspective of the RESPECTFUL counseling framework, it is vital that counselors conscientiously assess the ways in which the interaction of multiple factors of this framework influence their clients' and their own development. The following case scenario is presented to help counselors think about the ways in which the interplay of the first three factors in the RESPECTFUL counseling model (religious/spiritual identity, economic class background, and sexual identity) may affect David's psychologic development and daily functioning. The case scenario will also provide an opportunity for the counselor to examine how his or her own beliefs and attitudes affect the content and process of the counseling services that are offered to David.

Case Scenario 1

David is a 28-year-old, hard-of-hearing, Chinese gay male. He communicates well with his binaural hearing aids. For the past 2 years, he has been in a monogamous and satisfying relationship with Abe, who has normal hearing. David was raised in San Francisco by both hearing parents who have been married for nearly 30 years. His father is a minister and has always wanted David to be a minister since he was very young. This semester, David has been failing most of his classes with the exception of math and is in jeopardy of being kicked out of Bible College. David voluntarily seeks help from a counselor based, in large part, on the insistence of his partner, who thinks it would be useful for David to talk to a professional about his feelings of depression, guilt, anger, and sadness. David states that he does not want to be a minister and wants to change his major to accounting. David also shares the fact that he has not disclosed his sexual preference with his parents. Although he wants to talk with his parents about this aspect of his life, he is afraid of their reaction.

Counselors may consider how the interplay of three factors in the RESPECTFUL counseling model (religious/spiritual identity, economic class background, and sexual identity) have an impact on David's psychologic development and current daily functioning. A few questions that counselors may wish to explore include the following:

- How have David's religious upbringing, spiritual beliefs, and values influenced his life?
- How does the socioeconomic class in which David was raised influence his current way of thinking?
- How does David's sexual identity affect his psychologic disposition?

To examine how their own beliefs and attitudes affect how they react to the situation presented, counselors may consider the following questions:

- How do your religious/spiritual beliefs and values (or lack of) influence this counseling session?
- What biases do you bring from your economic background?
- Are you genuinely comfortable and confident working with persons with a gay lifestyle?

Psychologic Maturity

Counselors often work with clients who share common demographic characteristics (e.g., age, gender, socioeconomic, and cultural-racial backgrounds) but who appear to be very different psychologically. In these situations we may refer to one client as being "more psychologically mature" than another client who is the same age, identifies with the same cultural-racial reference group, and shares a similar sexual identity. Some descriptors that are commonly used by counseling professionals to describe this "immature" client include statements such as "he demonstrates limited impulse control in social interactions" or "she has a low capacity for self-awareness." Statements that are commonly used to describe "more mature" clients include "he is able to discuss his problems with much insight," "she is highly self-aware," and "he has developed a much broader range of interpersonal and introspective skills than many of the other clients with whom I am working."

Over the past 3 decades, our understanding of the developmental stages that individuals pass through as they mature psychologically has tremendously increased. Much of this understanding comes from the work of several cognitive-developmental psychologists who have presented numerous models that help explain the process of psychologic maturity. This includes the work of Piaget (1977) on cognitive development, Perry (1970) on ethical development, Kohlberg (1981) and Gilligan (1982) on moral development, Selman (1980) on social/interpersonal development, and Loevinger (1976) on ego development.

Cognitive-developmental theories view psychologic development as a process in which individuals move from simple to more complex ways of thinking about themselves and their life experiences. This movement can be traced along a set of invariant, hierarchical stages that reflect qualitatively different ways of thinking, feeling, and acting in the world (Sprinthall, Peace, & Kennington, 2001). According to Young-Eisendrath (1988), each developmental stage represents a uniquely different frame of reference for meaning-making. She goes on to identify that developmental stages "are not entirely dependent on chronological maturation.... Stages evolve with aging up to a point. However, when further development is not supported by environmental factors, a person may stop developing" (p. 71).

By assessing clients' levels of psychologic maturity, counselors are better positioned to more effectively design interventions that are tailored to accommodate their clients' unique personal strengths and meet their needs. It is also equally important that counselors reflect on their own psychologic development, because the therapeutic process can easily be undermined when practitioners are matched with clients who function at a more complex level of psychologic maturity than the level at which they operate.

ETHNIC/RACIAL IDENTITY

The term *ethnic* is derived from the Greek word meaning "nation." Thus the concept of *ethnic identity* refers to persons who identify with and are distinguished from others by the unique social-cultural characteristics, values, and traditions that have evolved within the nation-states in which they live or are descended from. Although individuals are commonly associated with large cultural-racial groups (i.e., African Americans, European Americans, or Native Americans), people commonly demonstrate strong personal identification with specific ethnic groups (e.g., Italian-Americans or Irish-Americans) whose values and traditions have had a substantial impact on their development and view of the world.

Historically, the term *race* has been used to connote both biologic and social differences. From a biologic perspective, people of different races have been classified into three major groups—Caucasoid, Mongoloid, and Negroid. Although these three categories have often been used to broadly distinguish racial differences in the past, they have recently been criticized as being misleading and superficial in terms of classifying persons according to phenotypic variations in skin color and other physical characteristics (Helms & Cook, 1999). The longstanding history in the United States of miscegenation (i.e., persons born to parents from different racial groups) has rendered such biologically based explanations of race relatively useless. The theory of miscegenation simply suggests that if everyone in the United States were able to accurately track their biologic lineage back in time, they would find that everyone in this country comes from a mixed racial blood lineage (Helms & Cook, 1999).

Another major problem associated with using externally manifested biologic traits to define racial differences is the compounding effect of within-group differences. Whereas researchers readily acknowledge that phenotypic differences (e.g., differences in skin color or hair texture) are apparent among many people in our society, there is actually greater genotypic variation (e.g., differences in a person's genetic makeup) among individuals who come from the same racial groups than among individuals who have been historically identified as belonging to different "racial groups" in this country (Allen & Adams, 1992; Helms & Cook, 1999; Zukerman, 1990).

Because scientific evidence clearly negates traditional definitions of race that are rooted in biologic–genetic differences, one may question the usefulness of thinking about human differences in racial terms at all. Given the ambiguity and confusion that surrounds the definition of the term *race* from a biologic perspective, it is reasonable to ask why this construct continues to be used to categorize people in our society.

To attempt to answer this question, Helms and Cook (1999) suggest that, rather than describing it in biologic terms, the word *race* can be more meaningfully defined as a social construction that is designed to assure that societal privileges are maintained among persons in certain racial groups in our society. This includes a range of privileges such as easier access to education and employment opportunities, health care resources, housing, and personal loans as well as differential sentencing for criminal acts and treatment by law enforcement personnel (Jones, 1997). When racial factors are considered, numerous researchers have reported that these and many other social privileges continue to be disproportionately bestowed among persons from middle and upper class white European backgrounds, particularly males, in our nation (Helms & Cook, 1999; Jones, 1997; Scheurich, 1993).

The various privileges, discrimination, and types of oppression that have been and continue to be bestowed among persons who are associated with different racial groups have a profound psychologic effect on the way individuals construct meaning of the world and themselves. Over the past 15 years, numerous researchers have shed light on the ways that persons from diverse groups develop a sense of identity that integrates reactions to one's racial background and experiences. The interested reader is encouraged to review Cross's (1995) model of black identity development as well as Helm's (1995) model of white identity development and her racial identity development framework for people of color to learn more about the different developmental statuses/stages and unique psychologic characteristics that distinguish persons who operate from the various levels of these developmental models.

Clearly, tremendous psychologic differences exist among persons within the same ethnic/racial group. This variation is commonly called *within-group* differences. Given the within-group variation that is notably manifested among persons from the same ethnic/racial groups, it is important that counselors develop the knowledge and skills necessary to accurately assess these important differences and respond to them in effective and respectful ways in various counseling settings. It is also very important that counselors understand how their own ethnic/racial experiences have affected their psychologic development, the way they construct meaning of the world, and the types of biases they have acquired toward others in the process.

CHRONOLOGIC/DEVELOPMENTAL CHALLENGES

In addition to the types of developmental changes that were discussed earlier in the psychologic maturity section, individuals also undergo systematic changes that are chronologically based. These age-related, developmental changes represent *chronological challenges* that individuals face at different points across the lifespan. Counseling practitioners are familiar with many of these challenges, because they represent the characteristics that we normally associate with infancy, childhood, adolescence, and adulthood.

Theorists who explain human development from a chronologic perspective are commonly called lifespan development (Craig, 1992; Havighurst, 1953; Shaffer, 1993) or maturational theorists (Erikson, 1968). Unlike the cognitive developmental theorists who look at a particular aspect of a person's psychologic maturity (e.g., intellectual, moral, and social development), lifespan development theorists examine an individual's growth from a more holistic perspective, which includes assessing the physical, cognitive, and psychologic changes that predictably occur at different times in an individual's life (D'Andrea & Daniels, 2001).

The specific changes that lifespan researchers have noted individuals normally undergo as they develop from infancy through adulthood include physical growth (i.e., bodily changes and the sequencing of motor skills), the emergence of different cognitive competencies (i.e., the development of perceptual, language, learning, memory, and thinking skills), and the manifestation of various psychologic skills (i.e., the ability to manage one's emotions and the demonstration of more effective interpersonal competencies) that occur over time (Shaffer, 1993). The ways in which individuals successfully negotiate the chronologic challenges that are commonly associated with infancy, childhood, adolescence, and adulthood largely determine the degree to which they develop a positive sense of self-esteem, lead productive lives, and experience personal satisfaction in life.

Human development researchers have greatly helped counselors refine their thinking regarding the unique challenges individuals face at different points across the lifespan. Pragmatically speaking, this knowledge enables practitioners to work more effectively with persons who face difficult chronologic challenges in their lives by implementing age-appropriate intervention strategies in different counseling settings. It also allows practitioners to be mindful of the unique challenges that they are likely to encounter when significant chronologic differences exist between them and their clients. D'Andrea and Daniels (1997) suggested that many young practitioners are likely to encounter major challenges in terms of gaining a high level of trust, respect, and sense of professional legitimacy when working with some clients who are much older than the counselors themselves.

The following case scenario is presented to highlight again the importance of considering multiple contexts of diversity that have an impact on both clients' and counselors' psychologic development. In this case scenario, counselors are encouraged to think about the ways in which the interplay of three factors contained in the RESPECTFUL counseling model (psychologic maturity, ethnic/racial identity, and chronologic challenges) may affect the content and process of the counseling services that are offered to Maria. Counselors should also consider how strengths and limitations associated with their age and their own cultural biases/preferences may influence their work with Maria.

Case Scenario 2

Maria is an extremely thin 12-year-old Filipino and Portuguese middle school-age girl. She was born deaf and was adopted when she was an infant by John and Mandy. Maria's adopted parents are both white, age 44 and 47 years, respectively. They are an upper middle-class family living in a predominately white neighborhood. Maria's parents admit that they spoil her, catering to her every whim. Because they are prominent business people, they have not had time to join the free sign language classes for parents of deaf children offered at the local church. They believe it is important for her to learn to communicate like other "normal" children her age. Although Maria has a history of struggling in school with her reading, lately her grades have dropped considerably; she isolates herself both at home and school, seems depressed all the time, and hardly eats. Her teacher refers Maria to the counseling office.

Counselors may consider ways in which the interplay of psychologic maturity, ethnic/racial identity, and chronologic challenges in the RESPECTFUL counseling model may have an impact on Maria's psychologic development and current daily functioning. A few questions that counselors may wish to explore include the following:

- What is Maria's level of psychologic development?
- In what ways is Maria psychologically different?
- What are some of the challenges that Maria encounters from a chronologic perspective?

To examine how their own beliefs and attitudes affect how they react to the situation presented, counselors may consider the following questions:

- Given your level of psychologic maturity, how comfortable are you with working with Maria?
- How may your cultural biases/preferences influence your work with Maria?
- What are the strengths and limitations of your age as you work with Maria?

TRAUMA AND OTHER THREATS TO ONE'S WELL-BEING

Trauma and threats to one's well-being are included in the RESPECTFUL counseling and development model to emphasize the complex ways in which stressful situations put people at risk of psychologic danger and harm. Such harm typically occurs when the stressors individuals experience in their lives exceed their ability to cope with them in constructive and effective ways. An individual's personal resources (coping skills, self-esteem, social support, and the personal power one derives from her or his cultural group) may be overtaxed when one is subjected to ongoing environmental stressors for extended periods. When individuals experience similar stressors for extended periods, they are commonly called a *vulnerable* or an *at-risk* group (Lewis, Lewis, Daniels & D'Andrea, 2003).

Counselors are often called upon to work with persons in various vulnerable, at-risk groups including poor, homeless, and unemployed people; adults and children in families undergoing divorce; pregnant teenagers; individuals with human immunodeficiency virus (HIV) infection or acquired immunodeficiency syndrome (AIDS); persons with cancer; and individuals who are victimized by various forms of ageism, racism, sexism, and cultural oppression. Although individuals in these vulnerable populations differ greatly from one another, they all routinely experience high levels of environmental stress that tax their personal resources and coping abilities. Heightened, prolonged, and historical stressors often result in more severe and adverse psychologic outcomes for many persons from oppressed cultural-ethnic-racial groups in our contemporary society. These stressors can and do result in traumatic life experiences underlying many of the intergenerational problems that are manifested among many persons from vulnerable groups in our nation (Salzman, 2001).

To be effective, counseling practitioners must accurately assess the different ways in which environmental stressors adversely affect clients' lives and develop intervention strategies that help to ameliorate these problems. Counselors who work with persons from diverse client populations must be knowledgeable of the ways in which intergenerational trauma is sustained over time and implement interventions that are intentionally designed to address such threats to clients' psychologic health and sense of well-being. It is also important for these practitioners to consider how various life stressors and traumatic events may have had a lasting impact on their own psychologic development.

FAMILY HISTORY AND INFLUENCE

The rapid cultural diversification of the United States includes an increasing number of families that are very different from the traditional notion of "family" that many counselors have historically used as a standard for determining "normal family life" and "healthy family functioning." The different types of families (e.g., single-female–headed families, blended families, extended families, and families headed by gay and lesbian parents) that counselors increasingly encounter in their work challenge them to reassess the traditional concept of the nuclear family that was used as a standard to which all other types of families were compared.

Increasingly, counselors will be pressed to understand the unique strengths that clients derive from these different family systems and implement counseling strategies that are intentionally designed to foster the healthy development of these diverse familial units. In addition to learning about the personal strengths that individuals derive from these different types of family systems, counseling practitioners are encouraged to assess biases and assumptions that they may have developed about family life as a result of their own unique family history and experiences. This is important, because when left unexamined, these biases and assumptions may adversely affect the counseling relationship with clients who come from families that are very different from that of the counselor's.

UNIQUE PHYSICAL CHARACTERISTICS

The RESPECTFUL counseling framework emphasizes the importance of being sensitive to the ways in which our society's idealized images of physical beauty have a negative impact on the psychologic development of many persons whose physical nature does not fit the narrow views of beauty that are fostered by our modern culture. McWhirter (1994) notes that "one of the most disheartening and frightening phenomena in our society is the relentless and all-consuming desire for physical beauty" (p. 203). This obsession is rooted in an idealistic image of individuals who are thin and muscular. In reality, few people match this idealistic image, and many experience reduced self-esteem and increased feelings of personal inadequacy as a result (McWhirter, 1994). In other instances, individuals with physical, mental, and emotional disabilities have also suffered from various forms of discrimination and stigmatization, whose genesis is rooted in misperceptions and stereotypes about physical beauty, ability, and health.

When working with clients whose unique physical characteristics may be a source of stress and dissatisfaction, counselors must reflect on the ways in which the idealized myth of physical beauty may have led them to internalize negative views and stereotypes about individuals who do not fit this myth. This is important, because when these sorts of internalized views go unchecked, they may lead to inaccurate assessments and misinterpretations of clients' psychologic dispositions. Also, when working with women and men whose psychologic development has been negatively affected by some aspect of their own unique physical nature, practitioners must be able to assist them to understand the ways in which gender role socialization contributes to irrational thinking about their own sense of self-worth.

LOCATION OF RESIDENCE AND LANGUAGE DIFFERENCES

The *location of one's residence* refers to the geographical region and setting where one resides. D'Andrea and Daniels (2001) identified five areas that many persons commonly refer to when talking about the major regions in the United States. These geographical areas are the northeastern, southeastern, midwestern, southwestern, and northwestern regions of our nation. They are distinguished by differences in climate patterns, geological terrain, occupations and industries available, and persons who reside there. Also, these geographical locations often are distinguished by their own unique subcultures that reflect different values, attitudes, and language or dialects that are commonly manifested by many individuals who reside in these areas.

Counseling practitioners are familiar with three major residential settings where many clients live: rural, suburban, and urban settings. As defined by the U.S. Bureau of the Census (2001), rural populations comprise people who live in towns of less than 2,500 inhabitants and in open country outside the closely settled suburbs of metropolitan cities. In contrast, urban areas comprise cities with 50,000 or more inhabitants (U.S. Bureau of the Census, 2001). When counseling practitioners work with persons who come from geographic regions or residential settings that are different from the ones in which they were raised, it is important that these practitioners reflect on the possible stereotypes and biases they may have developed about individuals who come from these different areas. This is particularly important when practitioners work with people who use a different dialect or language in interpersonal interactions. In the following case scenario, counselors are encouraged to consider the ways in which the interaction of Kathleen's daily stresses, family history, unique physical characteristics, and ecologic barriers that are contained in the RESPECTFUL counseling model, augmented with age-related hearing loss, might affect her psychologic well-being. As is the case with the other factors of the RESPECTFUL counseling model, self-reflection and assessment are also very important, because possible stereotypes and biases that counselors might have developed about their clients may lead to inaccurate assumptions and clinical interpretations within counseling settings.

Case Scenario 3

Kathleen is a 67-year-old, late-deafened, African-American woman who lives alone in a small, rural town in Georgia. Although Kathleen has had severe stomach problems and lost more than 20 pounds over the past 3 months, she ignored these physical developments, because she did not like going to the doctor. When she noticed blood in her stool, Kathleen was frightened and decided to see a physician. Cancer was diagnosed. She was so devastated that she was unsure whether her physician said surgery would help or whether and when she needed to begin chemotherapy. Kathleen refuses to share this diagnosis with anyone, because she fears that her daughter Angie will want her to leave her home to move in with Angie and her noisy three children in an apartment in New York, or, even worse, to move into a nursing home.

Counselors may consider ways in which the interaction of Kathleen's daily stresses, family history, unique physical characteristics, and ecologic barriers contained in the RESPECTFUL counseling model may have an impact on Kathleen's psychologic development and current daily functioning. A few questions that they may wish to explore include the following:

- Why are the identified stresses considered problematic for Kathleen?

- How have Kathleen's family dynamics affected her life?
- How have physical challenges influenced Kathleen's development psychologically?
- What different types of needs, stresses, and sources of support will Kathleen have if she moves to New York?

To examine how their own beliefs and attitudes affect how they react to the situation presented, counselors may consider the following questions:

- How do the daily stresses you experience impact your work with Kathleen?
- How have your family experiences influenced your comfort level in working with Kathleen?
- What are your biases regarding Kathleen's "physical-ness," and how do these biases impact your work with her?
- How may your residence preference influence your work with Kathleen?

CONCLUSION

The RESPECTFUL counseling model has practical utility to expand counselors' thinking about the various considerations that underlie a culturally competent approach to counseling practice. Recognizing that the components contained in this model do not represent an exhaustive list of all the factors that impact human development, practitioners and researchers should collaborate and continue to add to a better understanding of the multidimensionality of human development both personally and professionally.

REFERENCES

Allen, B. P., & Adams, J. Q. (1992). The concept "race": Let's go back to the beginning. *Journal of Social Behavior and Personality, 7,* 163–168.

American Counseling Association. (1996). *Code of ethics and standards of practice.* Washington, DC: Author.

American Psychological Association. (2002). *Ethical principles of psychologists and code of conduct.* Washington, DC: Author.

Atkins, B. J., & Wright, G. N. (1980). Three views: Vocational rehabilitation of Blacks. The statement, the response, the comment. *Journal of Rehabilitation, 46*(2), 40–49.

Bailey, J. M. (1996). Gender identity (pp. 71–93). In Savin-Williams, R. C. & Cohen, K. M. (Eds.), *The lives of lesbians, gays, and bisexuals: Children to adults.* Fort Worth, TX: Harcourt Brace.

Bowe, F. (1984). *U.S. Census and disabled adults.* Hot Springs, AR: University of Arkansas, Arkansas Services, Arkansas Rehabilitation Research and Training Center.

Commission on Rehabilitation Counselor Certification (2002). *Code of professional ethics.* Rolling Meadows, IL: Author.

Craig, G. J. (1992). *Human development* (6th ed.). Englewood Cliffs, NJ: Prentice Hall.

Cross, W. E., Jr. (1995). The psychology of nigrescence: Revising the Cross model (pp. 93–122). In Ponterotto, J. G., Casas, J. M., Suzuki, L. A., & Alexander, C. M. (Eds.), *Handbook of multicultural counseling.* Thousand Oaks, CA: Sage.

D'Andrea, M., & Daniels, J. (1997). RESPECTFUL counseling: A new way of thinking about diversity counseling. *Counseling Today, 40*(6), 30, 31–34.

D'Andrea, M., & Daniels, J. (2001). RESPECTFUL counseling: An integrative model for counselors (pp. 417–466). In Pope-Davis, D. & Coleman, H. (Eds.). *The interface of class, culture and gender in counseling.* Thousand Oaks, CA: Sage.

Erikson, E. (1968). *Identity: Youth and crisis.* New York: Norton.

Gilligan, C. (1982). *In a different voice: Psychological theory and women's development.* Cambridge, MA: Harvard University Press.

Havighurst, R. J. (1953). *Human development and education.* New York: Longman.

Helms, J. E. (1995). An update of Helm's white and people of color racial identity models (pp. 181–191). In Ponterotto, J. G., Casas, J. M., Suzuki, L. A., & Alexander, C. M. (Eds.), *Handbook of multicultural counseling.* Thousand Oaks, CA: Sage.

Helms, J. E., & Cook, D. A. (1999). *Using race and culture in counseling and psychotherapy: Theory and process.* Boston: Allyn & Bacon.

Jones, J. M. (1997). *Prejudice and racism* (2nd ed.). New York: McGraw Hill.

Kampfe, C. M. (1990). Communicating with persons who are deaf: Some practical suggestions for rehabilitation specialists. *Journal of Rehabilitation, 56,* 41–45.

Kampfe, C. M., & Smith, S. M. (1999). Late-onset hearing loss: Strategies for effective counseling. *Adultspan Journal, 1,* 32–49.

Kelly, E. W. (1995). *Spirituality and religion in counseling and psychotherapy: Diversity in theory and practice.* Alexandria, VA: American Counseling Association.

Kohlberg, L. (1981). *The philosophy of moral development.* San Francisco, CA: Harper & Row.

Lewis, J., Lewis, M., Daniels, J., & D'Andrea, M. (2003). *Community counseling: Empowerment strategies for a diverse society.* Pacific Grove, CA: Brooks/Cole.

Loevinger, J. (1976). *Ego development.* San Francisco, CA: Jossey-Bass.

McWhirter, E. H. (1994). *Counseling for empowerment.* Alexandria, VA: American Counseling Association.

Mindel, E. D., & Vernon, M. (1971). *They grow in silence: The deaf child and his family.* Silver Spring, MD: National Association of the Deaf.

Moore, C. L. (2001). Disparities in job placement outcomes among deaf, late-deafened, and hard of hearing consumers. *Rehabilitation Counseling Bulletin, 44*(3), 144.

Moore, C. L., & Schroedel, J. G. (2001). *A national profile of the vocational rehabilitation of Americans with hearing loss* (Tech Report). Little Rock, AR: Rehabilitation Research and Training Center for Persons who are Deaf and Hard-of-Hearing.

Patterson, J. B., Allen, T. B., Parnell, L., Crawford, R., & Beardall, R. L. (2000). Equitable treatment in the rehabilitation process: Implications for future investigations related to ethnicity. *The Journal of Rehabilitation, 66*(2), 14.

Perry, W. G. (1970). *Forms of intellectual and ethical development in the college years: A scheme.* New York: Holt, Rinehart, and Winston.

Piaget, J. (1977). *The development of thought: Equilibrium of cognitive structure.* New York: Viking.

Robertson, M. (1999). Counseling clients with acquired hearing impairment: Towards improved understanding and communication. *International Journal for the Advancement of Counseling, 21,* 31–42.

Salzman, M. B. (2001). Cultural trauma and recovery: Perspectives from terror management theory. *Trauma, Violence, & Abuse, 2,* 172–191.

Scheurich, J. J. (1993). Toward a discourse on white racism. *Educational Researcher, 22,* 5–10.

Selman, R. (1980). *The growth of interpersonal understanding: Developmental and clinical analysis.* New York: Academic Press.

Shaffer, D. R. (1993). *Developmental psychology: Childhood and adolescence* (3rd ed.). Pacific Grove, CA: Brooks/Cole.

Sprinthall, N. A., Peace, S. D., & Kennington, P. A. D. (2001). Cognitive-developmental stage theories for counseling (pp. 109–130). In Locke, D. C., Myers, J. E., & Herr, E. L., (Eds.), *The handbook of counseling.* Thousand Oaks, CA: Sage.

Sue, D. W., & Sue, D. (2003). *Counseling the culturally different: Theory and practice* (4th ed.). New York: John Wiley.

U.S. Bureau of the Census. (2001). *Geographic tools (Fact finder for the nation).* Washington, DC: U.S. Government Printing Office.

U.S. Surgeon General's Report. (2001). *Mental health: Culture, race, and ethnicity.* Department of Health and Human Services. Washington, DC: U.S. Government Printing Office.

Wilson, K. B. (2002). Exploration of VR acceptance and ethnicity: A national investigation, *Rehabilitation Counseling Bulletin, 45*(3), 168–169.

Young-Eisendrath, P. (1988). Making use of human development theories in counseling. In Hayes, R. & Aubrey, R. (Eds.), New directions for counseling and human development (pp. 66–84). Denver, CO: Love.

Zuckerman, M. (1990). Some dubious premises in research and theory on racial differences: Scientific, social, and ethical issues. *American Psychologist, 45,* 1297–1303.

SUBJECT INDEX

developmental challenges, 300–302
economic factors, 292–294
ethnic factors, 298–300
family factors, 303–304
language differences, 305–307
location of residence, 305–307
maturity factors, 296–297
racial factors, 298–300
sexual identity factors, 294–296
trauma, 302–303
unique physical images,
    accepting, 304–305
Retinal detachment, 86
Retinitis pigmentosa, 85
Retinopathy, diabetic, 86
Retinopathy, premature, 85
RNA, 59

S

SAT. *See* Speech awareness threshold
Semantic compaction, 226
Sensorineural hearing loss, 66–67
Serous, 134
Sexual orientation, 294–296
Speech
  audiometry, goals, 42–43
  audiometry, recognition threshold, 43–45
  output, 272–273
  recognition threshold, 43–44
Speech awareness threshold, 44–45
Spirituality, 291–292
Surgeon General's Report, 285–286

T

Tangible reinforcement operant conditioning
  audiometry, 42
TDD. *See* Telecommunication devices for the deaf
Tech Act. *See* Technology-Related Assistance
  for Individuals with Disabilities Act
Technology-Related Assistance for Individuals with
  Disabilities Act, 191, 212
Telecommunication devices for the deaf, 199, 201
Telephone typewriters, 199
Tests. *See also* Evaluations
  adults, 95–97
  children
    battery, 98–99
    behavior, 100
    environment, 100–101
    materials, 101, 103
    overview, 97–98
    reinforcers, 107, 109
  cognitive function, 123–126
  management1, 110–111
Tinnitus, age-associated, 119
TM. *See* Tympanic membrane
TROCA. *See* Tangible reinforcement operant condi-
  tioning audiometry
TTYs. *See* Telephone typewriters

Tympanic membrane
  in OM, 134
  perforated, 160
  status evaluation, 137
Tympanocentesis, 137
Tympanograms, normal, 49, 51
Tympanostomy, 147

V

VESID. *See* Vocational Educational Services for
  Individuals with Disabilities
Video-otoscopy, 33–34, 160
Viruses, 59
Vision skills, 217
Visual impairment. *See also* Eye
  aural testing
    adults, 95–97
    case histories, 95–96
    children, 97–100
    clinician's decorum, 93
    lighting, 96
    management, 110–111
    printed materials, 96–97
    response interpretation, 109–110
  causes, 79
  clinician-patient interaction, 93–94
  degrees, definition, 8
  epidemiology, 79
  hearing, normal, 111–113
  hearing, role of, 91–93
  hearing impairment
    assessment, 93–95
    counseling topics, 113–114
    deafblind, 114–115
    implications, 8–9
    relationship, 87–88
  impact, 78
Visual reinforcement audiometry, 40–41, 107
Vocabulary
  auditor scanning, 221
  expansion techniques, 224–226
  on manual systems, 227
  organizing, 223
  quantity, 224
  word completion, 225
  word prediction, 225
  word recognition ability, 45
Vocational Educational Services for Individuals with
  Disabilities, 278
VRA. *See* Visual reinforcement audiometry

W

Water Pik, 166–167
Within-group differences, 299–300
Words. *See* Vocabulary

Z

Zinc-Air batteries, 187

AUTHOR INDEX

	DATE DUE		